Issues in the Design
and
Evaluation of Medical Trials

Issues in the Design and Evaluation of Medical Trials

John M. Weiner, Dr. P.H.
Associate Professor of Medicine
University of Southern California
School of Medicine
Cottage A
2025 Zonal Avenue
Los Angeles, California 90033

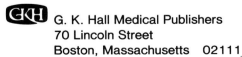 G. K. Hall Medical Publishers
70 Lincoln Street
Boston, Massachusetts   02111

G. K. Hall Medical Publishers
70 Lincoln Street
Boston, Massachusetts 02111

79 80 81 82 / 4 3 2 1

Weiner, John M.
Issues in the design and evaluation of
medical trials.

Includes bibliographical references and index.

1.   Human experimentation in medicine.   2.   Medicine,
Clinical—Research.   I.   Title.
R853.H8W44   619'.98   79-17519
ISBN 0-8161-2140-0

Issues in the Design and Evaluation of Medical Trials

Contents

Preface

Clinical research represents an integration of many procedures from the social, biological, and natural sciences. Critical examination of the spectrum of medical inquiries will reveal the full gamut of research activities. Understanding the processes involved in the integration of these investigative and cognitive functions may lead to further advances in creative behavior. The purpose of this book is to formalize this process by identifying, collecting, and organizing the elements and issues involved.

During the past thirty years, there have been significant advances in research methodology, many of them stimulated by multi-disciplinary collaboration. The anticipated barriers to communication were not realized in practice. Scientists engaged in mutual problem-solving could accomplish more than their colleagues working in relative isolation. In their productive fashion, these multi-disciplinary teams, by pooling their knowledge sets and by developing communication mechanisms, created the interfaces between the clinical, analytical, and communication sciences. These interfaces, while neither complete nor perfect, represent the methodology of interest in accomplishing the capture, evaluation, and utilization of information, or Information Processing. The list of contributors to this methodology is virtually endless and we acknowledge their enormous and significant efforts.

John M. Weiner

Issues in the Design and Evaluation of Medical Trials

Chapter 1

Research and Data

Training Clinical Specialists

Inherent in existing training programs in the various clinical specialties is the assumption that the student will also acquire expertise in clinical research as it is applied to the specialty. The emphasis, however, is on learning laboratory and/or clinical methods, and, consequently, there are limited opportunities to learn the techniques designed to manage the information derived as part of the research. While the purposes of these studies are to develop new information, the focus may be on a new technique or a new therapy rather than on the total research process. This is important in that, without a proper research structure to enhance awareness and understanding of the findings, the new method may be accepted or discarded without proper evaluation.

Priorities in the training of clinicians indicate that the present structure of clinical specialty programs is properly balanced. The major component of these programs is the acquisition of skills and knowledge relative to the set of methods and therapies used in the specialty. The continuing importance of critical evaluation provides students with the appropriate reinforcement of attitudes for pursuit of their own research programs. The volume of clinical material to be learned and applied, however, precludes opportunities to offer more than overviews to areas of information processing.

Typically, a clinical training program will include seminars in selected topics from biostatistics. Providing the trainee with clear-cut examples in the framework of that specialty is not easy. If the presentations are effective, the trainee will be exposed to selected issues associated with

1. study designs
2. such techniques as random allocation
3. statistical tests, e.g., Student t and chi-square.

Established clinical specialists who choose academic work soon learn that they are at a disadvantage. Training programs may provide the experiences necessary for learning appropriate methods and attitudes, and they may develop skills in matching scientific concepts to human problems. But the clinician is likely to lack both the skills and the knowledge needed to prepare, conduct, and report research.

Consultative Support

Academic institutions offer various forms of assistance to the would-be investigator. These organizational structures are described briefly in this section.

The simplest structure is the consultation service, which features data processing in such forms as card punching, verifying, listing, sorting, and collating. Numerical displays may be tabular. Statistical analyses, if performed, would feature tests of proportions or of frequencies. The methods used would be those described in elementary courses and textbooks.

A second organizational structure is the coordinating center. The statistical, computing, and data management personnel are organized to deal with specific clinical problems and to interact with clinical investigators in a study group. The structure may be designed to meet the study's needs as follows:

1. design the study to be conducted
2. train personnel
3. provide interim analyses reflecting accrual of patients, patient safety, and compliance with protocol
4. provide final analyses
5. assist in preparation of papers and reports.

The personnel involved are expected to produce methodological research as well as clinically oriented scientific findings.

A third structure can be found in the cooperative clinical groups studying the treatment of cancer. These groups study the many different and specific malignant diseases. The opportunities for interaction among the collaborating disciplines are more frequent in this setting. Different studies are likely to be in different phases—planning, conduct, analysis, or reporting—and the personnel are expected to produce new technologies relative to the entire clinical research process. The emphasis on diagnosis and treatment of multiple diseases stimulates review of those characteristics typical of both management and research.

Eisenhart, in discussing the role of a statistical consultant (1947), expressed his view as follows:

It was the advent of, study of, and experimentation with, first biological and later industrial material, subject to great and diverse forms of variation, that brought the need for statistical theory and methods of greater scope and effectiveness. And finally, given need, the required ideas and methods were not forthcoming until perspicacious men of statistical inclination and mathematical bent were given an opportunity to don overalls, or at least laboratory frocks, and work side-by-side with those who were grappling with the problems to be solved.

The Patient Management Protocol

Guidelines for each disease type and medical specialty are useful in describing the appropriate approaches to evaluate and care for patients with a given disease. These guidelines, which are most often found in review articles, represent an underlying set of procedures, involving information segments and decision-making criteria. As such, the standards for the care of a patient with a given disease can be designated as a management protocol. The specific areas are

1. identification
2. documentation of disease
3. extent of disease
4. function tests
5. treatments
6. adverse effects
7. status.

Examples of the record types used in cancer are given in Table 1.1.

The identification data convey sociological, cultural, and economic overtones associated with such items as name, residence, occupation, age, sex, and ethnic affiliation. These data are obtained primarily to provide personal identification, but a researcher can expect relationships to natural history and epidemiological findings. The data base created here is then used for later reference.

Documentation of the disease contains those findings which assist the physician in identifying the disease type. The data included depend upon these criteria:

1. the disease
2. the patient's past history (previous findings)
3. the availability of diagnostic procedures in the institution
4. financial considerations
5. community standards of performance.

The data contained in the extent of disease segment of the protocol describe the presenting impact of the disease. Depending on these findings, the general associations from natural history data are modified to account for specific host-disease interactions.

Table 1.1
Record Types

A. Identification

Direct Access Alpha Record
  Name: *Last, First, Initial*
  Hospital ID Number
  Address: *Number, Street, City, Zip Code*
  Telephone: *Area Code, Number*

Direct Access Numeric Record
  Date Referral
  Date Consult
  Reason for Request: *Diagnosis, Treatment,*
    Transfer
  First Symptom
    Date
  First Sign
    Date
  Evidence Malignancy: *Physical Exam, X-ray,*
    Laboratory, Tissue
  Recommendation: *Diagnosis, Treatment,*
    Transfer
    Accept: *In, Out*
    Reject
  Date Decision / Recommendation
  Referring Diagnosis
  Oncology Diagnosis
    Date Established
  Age
  Sex
  Race

Master Record
  Name: *Last, First, Initial*

B. Documentation of Disease

Scan Report
  Date
  Site
  Size
  Extent

X-Ray Report
  Date
  Site
  Size
  Extent

Special Laboratory Study
  Date
  Name of Test
  Finding *(Numeric Entry)*

Angiography
  Date
  Site
  Size
  Extent

Special Study
  Date
  Name of Test
  Finding *(Numeric Entry)*

Bone Marrow Report
  Date
  Site
  Percent Fat
  Percent "Normal" Cells
  Percent "Abnormal" Cells
  Diagnosis

Mammography Report
  Date
  Location
  Finding *(Numeric Entry)*
  Size
  Extent

Biopsy Report
  Date
  Site
  Histology
  Diagnosis

Autopsy
  Date
  Primary
  Metastatic Distribution

C. Extent of Disease

Sites of Involvment
  Location*
  Date First Diagnosed
  Primary / Metastatic
  Date Report
    Sub-location*
    Side
    Size
    Extent
    Evidence: *Physical Exam, X-ray, Scan,*
      Laboratory, Tissue

*Sites of Involvement (Location)

  Skin
  Bone
  Muscle
  Periph. Nervous System
  Cardiovascular
  Bone Marrow
  Nodes
  Spleen
  CNS:
    Nervous
    Mesenchymal
    Meninges
    Pituitary / Pineal Body
    Eyes & Adnexia

Table 1.1 Cont.
Record Types

C. Extent of Disease

Ear
Jaws-Teeth
Oral Cavity & Pharynx
Upper Respiratory Tract
Lower Respiratory Tract
Pleura
Diaphragm
Esophagus
Breast
Digestive System:
  Stomach
  Intestine
  Rectum
  Liver, Gallbladder
  Ascites
  Pancreas
Urogenital-Adrenal:
  Adrenal
  Kidney, Renal Pelvis, Ureter
  Urinary Bladder
Male Sex Organs:
  Prostate
  Testis
  Other
Female Sex Organs:
  Vulva, Vagina, Uterus
  Cervix
  Endomyometrium
  Pelvic Structures
  Ovary
  Fallopian Tubes

D. Function Tests

Clinical Laboratory
  Date
  BUN
  Creatinine
  Uric Acid
  Total Bilirubin
  Direct Bilirubin
  SGOT
  SGPT
  Alkaline Phosphatase
  Albumin
  Acid Phosphatase
  Alpha-Feto Protein
  HBSAG
  CA + +
  Blood Sugar
  Urine Protein
  Urine White Blood Cell Count
  Urine Red Blood Cell Count
  CEA

Hemogram
  Date
  Platelets

  HCT
  HGB

White Blood Cell Count
Percent Segs (PMN)
  Bands
  Meta
  Myelo
  Pro
  Blasts
  Lymph
  Mono
  Eos
  Baso
  Plasma

E. Treatments

Prescriptions
  Date
  Agent
  Dose / M^2
  Dose / KG
  Schedule
  Route
  M^2 *(Body Surface Area)*
  Weight
  Height

Surgery
  Date
  Purpose: *Dx, Rx, Palliative*
  Site
  Result

X-ray Therapy
  Site
  Date Start
  Date Report *(Stop)*
  Total Rads
  Tumor Responsive: *Yes, No*

Supportive Therapy
  Type
  Date
  Dose
  Reason

Hormonal Therapy
  Type
  Purpose *Add., Abl.*
  Date Start
  Date End
  Tumor Responsive: *Yes, No*
  Weight
  Height
  M^2

Immunotherapy
  Type
  Date Start
  Date Report *(Stop)*
  Dose

Table 1.1 Cont.
Record Types

E. Treatments	G. Status (continued)

E.   Treatments

Tumor Responsive: *Yes, No*
Weight
Height
M²

Chemotherapy
   Type
   Date Start
   Date Report *(Stop)*
   Dose
   Tumor Responsive: *Yes, No*
   Weight
   Height
   M²

F.   Toxicities and Complications

Date
Pain
Nausea
Vomiting
Diarrhea

Oral
Nervous System
Infection
Bleeding
Respiratory
Cardiac
Skin
Hair
GU
Temperature
Other

G.   Status

Status Record—Study
   Study Number
   Date Started
   Date Stopped
   Status: *On, Off, No Study*

Status Record—Survival
   Date
   Status: *Live, Dead, Lost*

The fourth segment, involving function tests, is more directly tied to the search-review process. These tests are often important in staging insights and in describing concomitant problems. Many of the function tests can be chosen to describe the patient's overall health status. These tests are additionally useful in providing a baseline description of the patient *prior* to the administration of specific and supportive therapies. As such, function test results serve to provide data to help the clinician continue to separate the adverse effects of the therapy from the progression of the disease.

The fifth information segment describes the therapy. This section documents the interactions among the various specialists managing the disease. As a result, detailed data sets should be available.

The sixth section includes data related to the adverse effects of therapy, or the toxicities and the adverse effects of the disease process, or the complications.

The last information segment documents the surveillance of the patient's status through time. The process used to assess status will depend on the type of problem considered. For example, status relative to toxicity or complications would involve repeated use of function tests, while status relative to disease control would involve both function tests and assays listed under the documentation of and extent of disease sections. Status relative to survival may represent either the usual processes or investigative efforts with methods different from those included in the outline, such as the "tracing of missing persons."

Information is generated as a result of providing care, and the outline suggests a close association between the data obtained and the adherence to a management protocol. In a given clinical setting, close compliance with the protocol would, by definition, be considered quality care. Documentation of quality is reflected by the adequacy, timeliness, and accuracy of data recording. The relationship between the management protocol and the quality of care should be implicit in the data gathering, recording, analysis, and reporting. This is comprehensive data management.

Issues in Data Management

Data management is best defined as a series of tasks and procedures appropriate to the capture, translation, and communication of information. The scope of the information processing is related to the reasons for instituting the process. Reasons frequently cited are

1. Need for quality assurance. Documentation of patient management, as described by the observations and measurements associated with the management.
2. Need for historical data. This requires developing a mechanism for the storage, retrieval, and display of patient data associated with diagnostic, current therapy, and outcome measures.
3. Need for current data. This mandates development of a process for the ongoing, current capture, editing, storage, retrieval, analyses, decision-making, and reporting of the individual patient's data as well as of data representing groups of patients.

The purpose of the designed data management system is to provide the desired information at the lowest cost when it is needed. The following examples of data recording and analysis illustrate the interrelationships between patient and data management.

Format in Data Recording

Data items related to the recognition and description of angina follow.

Current Format

Angina—may circle any set of numbers

00 = none

01 = symptoms with stress

02 = activity limited by angina

03 = angina at rest

04 = atypical angina

05 = chest pain—probably not angina

06 = recent onset—one month

07 = crescendo angina or impending myocardial infarction (M.I.) —mild

08 = crescendo angina or impending myocardial infarction (M.I.) —severe

09 = unknown

The entries under Current Format represent a recording structure that can be found in numerous forms. The numbers used were selected to insure uniqueness to each characteristic. While each is unique, the items are not mutually exclusive and the number scheme is not suitable for analyzing multiple characteristics, even though the instructions for recording the data do include multiple entry possibilities.

The items were rearranged as shown in the Suggested Format.

Suggested Format

Angina   No data (quality control) ___

1—at rest (Yes = 2; No = 1)

2—with stress? (Yes = 2; No = 1)

3—activity limited by angina? (Yes = 2; No = 1)

4—atypical angina? (Yes = 2; No = 1)

5—chest pain—not angina? (Yes = 2; No = 1)

6—crescendo angina? (No = 1; Mild = 2; Severe = 3)

7—recent onset? ____ (YYMMDD)
                date

The questions associated with the presence and description of angina are now isolated from one another, so that any combination can be recorded and analyses devised to evaluate the different patterns.

Missing Data

The first question in Suggested Format illustrates a common problem. The failure to find data in the primary records may be because of

1. the absence of angina and the appropriate absence of a record, or
2. the presence of angina, but the failure to enter the data into the primary record.

If the first reason were known to be true, the patients with or without angina could be identified for subsequent scientific analyses. If the second reason were true, there are obvious flaws in the procedures used to effect accurate and complete reporting. This is a quality control problem.

First Analytical Questions

Frequently the first level of analysis involves the counting of attributes. In graphic form, the display may appear as shown in Figure 1.1. The vertical

Fig. 1.1.
Graphic Display of Angina Data.

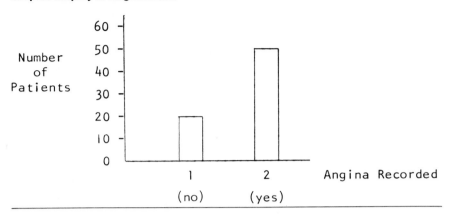

scale might be the "number of patients" or the "percent of patients." The horizontal scale is used to depict the numerical codes for the presence or absence of angina. The heights of the bars denote the numbers of patients in the subgroups.

The same information could be provided as shown in Table 1.2. The columns, from left to right, represent the value of the variate considered, the number of patients with the value, the percent of patients with the value, the cumulative number of patients, and the cumulative percent of patients.

Table 1.2
Tabular Display of Angina Data

Variate	Frequency	Percent	Cumulative Frequency	Cumulative Percent
1 (no)	20	28.6	20	28.6
2 (yes)	50	71.4	70	100.0

Second Analytical Questions
Frequency analyses of individual variates are a primary form of analysis. Coupling these variates leads to relationship questions and a basic analytical format used in screening data to find "clues" for further investigation. A variety of statistical models could be employed. For example, the 2 $\times$ 2 table can be used to explore the association between two variates when both are depicted at two levels (Table 1.3). The analysis in Table 1.3 includes as A_+ and A_- the information available from Table 1.2.

Table 1.3
Example of Two by Two (2 × 2) Table Format

		Angina		
		Yes	No	Total
	Yes	a	b	0_+
Other	No	c	d	0_-
Attribute	Total	A_+	A_-	T

a = Number of patients with both angina and the other attribute.
b = Number of patients without angina but with the other attribute.
c = Number of patients with angina but without the other attribute.
d = Number of patients without either angina or the other attribute.
A_+ = Total number of patients with angina.
A_- = Total number of patients without angina.
0_+ = Total number of patients with the other attribute.
0_- = Total number of patients without the other attribute.
T = Total number of patients studied.

Priority Assignment
The large number of 2 × 2 tables represent the pairing of the data items.
The number of tables depends upon the number of variates used:

$$\tfrac{1}{2} n(n - 1)$$

where n = the number of variates. For example, with 30 variates, there
would be

$$\tfrac{1}{2}(30)(29) = (15)(29) = 435 \text{ tables.}$$

Because of the large number of tables possible, a priority scheme should
be established. This might be done by asking the following: Assuming a
highly significant statistical association between two variates, would that
association be important clinically in terms of

1. a new finding never before reported?
2. a new finding suggested by previous data, i.e., new measurements
   used which are more specific but confirm previously reported less
   specific data?
3. a newer finding confirming reports by others; importance stems from
   the newness of the findings?
4. an older finding confirming previous reports; significance is in quality
   assurance of the data rather than the scientific issues?
5. an older finding of little interest whether it confirms or refutes previous reports; of no importance for either quality assurance or
   science?

With the importance of the findings identified and ranked, the corresponding analyses represent the significant and interesting ones to consider. A priority approach is superior to the mechanical generation of analyses. The former provides scientifically satisfying results and is more economical.

Preconceived Analyses
This approach establishes a set of scientifically interesting questions and assigns to each a priority for investigation.

In this exercise, a variate is selected to most clearly represent the patient's outcome relative to the diagnostic or therapeutic process. For example, such a variate might be Time to Death. Each patient can be characterized by this variate, which begins at some critical date (i.e., time first seen, time of first diagnosis) and terminates with date of death. The termination date for survivors can be the date last known to be alive.

Assuming the Time to Death variate to be true, other variates can be chosen to represent the patient's initial condition and the therapeutic process.

Once the entry variates are identified, the effects of treatment on the subgroups of patients with different entry patterns can be assessed. For example, consider that two groups of patients have been identified using pretherapy data. One group has severe angina, hypertension, and transmural myocardial infarction. This group may have a much shorter survival period when compared to a normotensive group with no angina or transmural myocardial infarction. A graphic description of this possibility is shown in Figure 1.2.

The curves shown describe the percent of hypothetical patients alive at

Fig. 1.2.
Natural History and Survival Data.

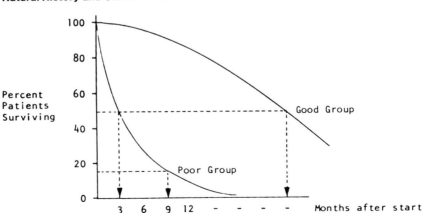

each month following entry into the study. The "poor" group's experience is indeed poor, with 50% of the patients alive at 3 months, 15% alive at 9 months, and 1% alive at 18 months. The "good" group's experience is significantly better. (The statistical assessment has suggested that there will be a very low probability that the two observed curves will represent a situation of equal survival experience.) Fifty percent of the patients are alive at 24 months and 15% are alive at 36 months, when the study ends. Longer surveillance is not shown, since in this example the patients had not been studied longer than the 36 months.

This result can now be assessed to determine the effectiveness of treatment. Assume that the "poor" group can be divided into two segments, one receiving effective treatment (about 25% of the patients) and the other receiving minimal or no treatment (about 75% of the patients). The "poor" group's survival curve represents the combined survival experiences of the two treatment segments. The more specific survival curves appear in Figure 1.3.

Note that the survival curve for the effective-treatment segment is close to that of the "good" group, and that the curve for the minimal-treatment segment is close to that of the whole "poor" group. The difference between the effective-treatment segment and the minimal-treatment segment is significant. The difference between the "good" group and the effectively treated "poor" segment is not statistically significant. This lack of difference is clinically important.

Structure of the Variate
The variate can, by its structure, guide and limit the analytical potential.

Fig. 1.3.
Treatment Influence on Natural History.

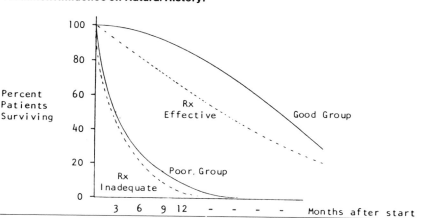

The Binomial Variate

This variate is theoretically the simplest in format and consists of *two* identifiable conditions, each of which can be assigned a *name,* for example:

1. survival status: living; dead

2. health status: well; sick

In addition to general-assessment functions, the binomial variate approach can be used to depict results of sophisticated laboratory issues, for example:

1. enzyme present?   yes; no

2. DNA repaired?   yes; no

In either description, the product for analysis is the same, i.e., a number is assigned to each condition with the agreement that the number is a pseudonym for the original name. Number pairs used frequently are: 0,1 and/or 1,2.

Binomial variates may be effectively used to develop a series of numbers depicting different situations, for example:

1. angina: yes; no

2. hypertension: yes; no

3. acute MI: yes; no

Assign 0 to No and 1 to Yes. Consider the sums of the three variates as shown in Table 1.4.

With the rule of simple summation, the presence of one of the conditions is indistinguishable from the presence of some other one because each single condition has the value 1, all double conditions have the value 2, and

Table 1.4
Simple Sum of Three Attributes

Angina	+	Hypertension	+ Acute M.I.	= Total
0		0	0	0
1		0	0	1
0		1	0	1
0		0	1	1
1		1	0	2
1		0	1	2
0		1	1	2
1		1	1	3

so forth. This rule simply totals the number of conditions found in the patient.

An alternative rule from binary arithmetic would be to arrange the conditions in order and assign the first the value 2^0, the second the value 2^1, and the third the value 2^2. The symbols stand for the number of times 2 is multiplied by itself, i.e., $2^2 = 2 \times 2$. Multiply the patient's values (the 0 or 1 for each condition) by the appropriate value of 2 (see Table 1.5).

Table 1.5
Summation Using Binary Arithmetic

Angina 2^2	+	Hypertension 2^1	+	Acute MI 2^0	=	Total
0		0		0		0
0		0		1		1 *
0		1		0		2
0		1		1		3
1		0		0		4
1		0		1		5
1		1		0		6
1		1		1		7

*Total $= 0 \times 2^2 + 0 \times 2^1 + 1 \times 2^0$
$= 0 \times 4 + 0 \times 2 + 1 \times 1$
($n^0 = 1$ where n = any value)

This summation process yields a scale of integers ranging from 0 to the total $2^p - 1$, where p = number of binomial variates used. In this example, $p = 3$, and the largest value is $2^3 - 1 = (2 \times 2 \times 2) - 1 = 8 - 1 = 7$.

With a summation rule using binary arithmetic and binomial variates, numerical scales may be developed describing subgroups of patients with varying, and increasing, combinations of conditions. The original order of the variates is crucial to the interpretation of the number scale. In Table 1.5, this is demonstrated by the values 3 and 4. The value 3 was generated by the presence of both hypertension and acute MI. The value 4 was dictated by the presence of angina only. The value 4 could be assigned to any other single condition which was placed as the third variate in the summation list.

The Multinomial Variate
This structure consists of *more* than two identifiable conditions, each of which is assigned a numerical pseudonym. Ideally, the numerical assignment should correspond with the clinical ordering of the conditions. In gen-

eral, the multinomial variate provides less flexibility than the binomial variate in describing clinical conditions. Its use should be restricted to applications where the number assignment can be easily justified.

The Continuous Variate

The continuous variate measurement offers the greatest flexibility in terms of analytical potential. The scale may be divided into intervals to represent either the binomial or multinomial situations. In addition, a larger number of computational models may be readily applied to the original variate.

This variate is used to develop such summary values of the data set as the mean, the standard deviation, and the correlation coefficient. In addition, summary patterns integrating—with appropriate weighting—original variate values may be computed. These patterns are useful in exploring the relationships among variates in different patient subgroups.

Integrating Clinical Research and Patient and Data Management

The medical trial is the process that integrates procedures of patient care and of data management in order to answer medical questions. To answer medical questions by this process, emphasis in the patient care protocol must be modified to reflect the new data needs.

Translating standard patient care in the clinical research protocol requires specific procedures. These procedures will be presented in subsequent chapters. In addition to the discussion of methodology, the logistics of planning and evaluating medical research will be illustrated. If these creative elements can be dissected into simpler components, learning should become easier.

Chapter 2

Patient Management and Decision Models

Introduction

Attempts to describe and formalize the functions performed by the health care provider have been presented in a number of distinguished medical journals. Dudley, in 1968, in describing approaches to formalizing the diagnostic process stated:

It can be argued that all that I have written here merely formalises well-known and self-evident truths. This is so, but formal statements are a necessary preliminary to the use of computers and the attraction of these processes is that the first two (pay-off and heuristics) and the dissective aspects of pattern recognition can all be handled by computer techniques. . . . the most important thing for the physician as a teacher to realise is that with or without the intervention of the computer the techniques described apply in clinical practice. . . . until the advent of the computer and the logical activity it demands we have not endeavoured to understand our actions in the diagnostic situation. It is scarcely surprising that the student is confused when, with his background of training in the formal deductive logic of the scientific laboratory, he sees the clinician adopt gaming, goal seeking, and pattern recognition. He is both confused and frustrated when in reply to his question—"why do you behave in such a way?"— the answer has been in the past, "this is the art of medicine." . . . if the techniques we use are analysable there exists the opportunity of creating repetitive educational situations which should lead to the more rapid attainment of diagnostic skills.

Formalizing behavioral methods and decision-making processes and making them reproducible are necessary for the introduction of scientific method into the clinical milieu. It is also important to recognize that the clinical setting is complex and requires sophisticated methodology to describe it properly. This chapter will present the ideas now called *clinical decision analysis*. This approach is of interest because it is used to depict the "ideal" clinical decision process and to evaluate the efficacy of observed processes. With growing emphasis on limiting cost and the increasing importance of malpractice considerations, clinical decision analysis should be reviewed by all care providers, whether or not research is involved (Taylor 1976).

The analytical approach incorporates flow diagram ideas from computer technology, logical manipulations, and Boolean algebra, integrated with clinical concepts pertinent to the disease process under consideration.

Logic and Logical Operations

In its simplest meaning, *logic* is *reason*. According to Webster's Collegiate Dictionary, logic "is the science that deals with the canons and criteria of validity of inference and demonstration" (Webster 1977). The term *statements* as used in this book refers to other observations based on fact or conclusions about these observations. Each statement may therefore be described as true (T) or false (F). These statements may be referred to by the alphabetical notation A, B, C, and so on, or numerically by 1, 2, 3, and so on. Both are a shorthand convenience. The designated symbol is a substitute for reiterating the statement each time it is used. When there are many statements, designation numbers are more convenient to use than letters.

Consider this example:

Statement A is:

	True	False	
Statement B is: True	Both are true	A is false B is true	B is true ignoring A
False	A is true B is false	Both are false	B is false ignoring A

All T and F possibilities for a group of n statements may also be shown in tabular form. The statements form the horizontal rows and their possible true and false combinations are denoted by T or F in the vertical columns. Such tables (called truth tables) have n rows and 2^n columns. Representing the symbols, T and F, by 1 and 0 respectively, provides a computational convenience when doing logical arithmetic.

Logical addition involves compound statements of the form—*either* A *or* B is true, or both are true—and would be denoted as (A + B). A compound statement involves two conditions. As an example consider the statements

A—the object is a dog
B— the object is black

The truth table is

Statements	Combinations of A and B			
A	T	F	T	F
B	T	T	F	F

or, using designation numbers, it is

Statements	Designation Numbers			
A	1	0	1	0
B	1	1	0	0

(A + B) would then have 1 1 1 0 as a designation number. This implies either that both A and B are true or that A or B is true. The verbal translation is that the object is either a dog, black, or a black dog. This is called *logical addition* and its rules can be stated like this:

$1 + 1 = 1$
$0 + 1 = 1$
$1 + 0 = 1$
$0 + 0 = 0.$

Another compound statement is denoted by (A · B). Both A *and* B are true only if A is true and B is true. The result is obtained by *logical multiplication.* The numerical rules are

$1 \times 1 = 1$
$1 \times 0 = 0$
$0 \times 1 = 0$
$0 \times 0 = 0.$

Logical multiplication is used when an outcome requires the presence of two independent variables. It can be applied to such compound statements as: both A *and* B are true only if A is true and B is true (A · B). This is another tabular way of presenting the logical multiplication of conditions A and B. Note that only when A is T and B is T does the outcome 1 occur.

Statement	*1*	*2*	*3*	*4*
A	T	F	T	F
B	T	T	F	F
A	1 (Dog)	0 (Not Dog)	1 (Dog)	0 (Not Dog)
B	1 (Black)	1 (Black)	0 (Not Black)	0 (Not Black)
(A · B)	1 (Black Dog)	0 —	0 —	0 —

Logical negation of statement A is obtained by switching all 0s to 1s and all 1s to 0s in the original designation number. That is, reversing the original designations

Statement

A	(Dog)	(Not Dog)	(Dog)	(Not Dog)
	1	0	1	0
$\overline{A}$	(Not Dog)	(Dog)	(Not Dog)	(Dog)
	0	1	0	1

The negation of A is denoted by placing a bar over A. The negation of B is $\overline{B}$.

Statement

B	(Black)	(Black)	(Not Black)	(Not Black)
	1	1	0	0
$\overline{B}$	(Not Black)	(Not Black)	(Black)	(Black)
	0	0	1	1

The compound statements would be

Compound Statement

$(A + B)$	1	1	1	0
	either (Black Dog) *or* (Black) *or* (Dog)			
$(\overline{A + B})$	0	0	0	1
				(*Neither* Black nor Dog)
$(A \cdot B)$	1	0	0	0
	(Black Dog)			
$(\overline{A \cdot B})$	0	1	1	1
		(Not Black)	(Not Dog)	(Neither Dog nor Black)

Complex logical statements may be expressed in a relatively numerical form by rearranging the designation numbers. For example, consider

Statement	Designation Number			
	1	*2*	*3*	*4*
$(\overline{A} + \overline{B})$	0	1	1	1
$(A + B)$	1	1	1	0
$(\overline{A} + \overline{B}) \cdot (A + B)$	0	1	1	0

The designation numbers represent the result or outcome. The interpretation of this result is that the compound multiplicative statement will be true if either of two conditions holds. These specific conditions are symbolized by the statements made in columns 2 and 3 of the original logical basis for A and B. These were

Statement	Designation Number			
	1	*2*	*3*	*4*
A: Object is a dog	1	0	1	0
B: Object is black	1	1	0	0

$(\overline{A} + \overline{B}) \cdot (A + B)$ will therefore be true if either the object is not a dog and black as shown by designation numbers 0 and 1 in column 2, or if the object is a dog and not black as represented by numbers 1 and 0 in column 3. The complex statement will be false under the other two conditions.

Two statements are identical only if *both* have the same designation number. This is called *logical identity.* Logical identity permits complex statements to be recognized as having the same or different meanings. For example, consider these two complex statements $(\overline{A} + \overline{B}) \cdot (A + B)$ and $(A \cdot \overline{B}) + (\overline{A} \cdot B)$.

The designation number for $(\overline{A} + \overline{B}) \cdot (A + B)$ is 0 1 1 0. The designation number for $(A \cdot \overline{B}) + (\overline{A} \cdot B)$ is also 0 1 1 0.

Statement	Designation			
A	1	0	1	0
B	1	1	0	0
$\overline{A}$	0	1	0	1
$\overline{B}$	0	0	1	1
$(A \cdot \overline{B})$	0	0	1	0
$(\overline{A} \cdot B)$	0	1	0	0
$(A \cdot B) + (\overline{A} \cdot B)$	0	1	1	0

The two compound statements $(\overline{A} + \overline{B}) \cdot (A + B)$ and $(A \cdot \overline{B}) + (\overline{A} \cdot B)$ are therefore alternative forms of the same statement.

Constrained Logical Basis
As the number of statements, n, increases in size, the number of columns, 2^n, grows even faster (e.g., two statements, $2^2 = 4$ columns; three statements, $2^3 = 8$ columns). Many combinations, while logically possible, are not probable or necessary. These constraints eliminate many columns. Moreover, by using the identity concept and considering the fact that any 2^n column designation number may be obtained as a sum of logi-

cal products, the simplest set of statements and corresponding columns may be retained.

This implies that procedures (equipment, methods) representing specific elemental statements may be combined and treated as if the result were also an elemental statement. Higher order statements may be retained. The simpler ones, now redundant, would be removed.

Symptom-Diagnosis Tables

Logical operations provide a means of exploring and depicting relationships between symptoms and diagnoses. A table which relates every possible combination of symptoms to diagnoses may be constructed. This table will contain a list of possible symptoms and a list of possible diagnoses. For n symptoms and m causes, there will be $n + m$ rows and 2^{n+m} columns. This will permit various combinations and comparisons.

To illustrate these possibilities, two symptoms and two diagnoses are shown in Table 2.1. The possible combinations are shown in 16 columns. The combination of the two symptoms, $S(1)$ and $S(2)$, produce four possible symptom complexes, s^i, $i = 1, 2, 3, 4$, which are shown in the second row. The blend of two diagnoses, $D(1)$ and $D(2)$, produces four complexes, d_j, $j = 1, 2, 3, 4$. Upper case letters, S or D, refer to single symptoms or diagnoses; lower case letters, s or d, refer to complexes or combinations of symptoms and/or diagnoses.

Each column represents possible combinations of diagnoses and symptoms that could occur. Column 1 describes the result of the absence of symptoms $S(1)$ and $S(2)$, and diagnoses $D(1)$ and $D(2)$. Column 12 presents the situation in which both symptoms and diagnosis $D(2)$ are available. Columns 4, 8, and 16 show the presence of both symptoms

Table 2.1
Symptom-Diagnosis Complex

Column Number Superscript i	Symptom Complex s^i															
	1 s^1	**2** s^2	**3** s^3	**4** s^4	**5** s^1	**6** s^2	**7** s^3	**8** s^4	**9** s^1	**10** s^2	**11** s^3	**12** s^4	**13** s^1	**14** s^2	**15** s^3	**16** s^4
S(1)	0	1	0	1	0	1	0	1	0	1	0	1	0	1	0	1
S(2)	0	0	1	1	0	0	1	1	0	0	1	1	0	0	1	1
D(1)	0	0	0	0	1	1	1	1	0	0	0	0	1	1	1	1
D(2)	0	0	0	0	0	0	0	0	1	1	1	1	1	1	1	1
Diagnosis Complexes Subscript j	d_1				d_2				d_3				d_4			

1. without either D(1) or D(2) being present
2. with diagnosis D(1) present
3. with both diagnoses present.

Table 2.1 illustrates the importance of restricting the focus to significant combinations; it is unproductive to consider all possible combinations. Limiting the analysis to those combinations which actually occur allows for nonrandom decision-making.

Constraints are chosen to be congruent with actual behavior and to permit the use of a sequential approach. This sequence will employ convenient and less expensive tests in preference to difficult and costly ones. The search for constraints will therefore be governed by simple observations or tests before more definitive and diagnostic ones. Table 2.2, a constraint table, contains 14 symptom possibilities and 8 diagnostic possibilities. The symptom-diagnosis possibilities have been confined to 16 columns. This table ranks the diagnostic tests in terms of difficulty and cost.

Table 2.3 illustrates the elimination of symptom-diagnosis columns by finding compound statements with zero values for those columns. Alternatively, the search may focus on those compound statements giving symptom-diagnosis complexes with values of one. For example, the history items, S(2) and S(3), when combined as a logical multiplicative compound statement, eliminate columns 12 through 16. The physical findings involving S(4), S(5), and S(6) eliminate columns 1, 2, 10, and 11.

The significance of the blood tests, S(7) through S(12), is less obvious and initial tests might be chosen to conform with equal numbers of zeros and ones in the columns of interest. As seen, S(9) and S(12) have 4 ones and 3 zeros; S(10) has 3 ones and 4 zeros. The minimum number of tests to choose would be

$\log_2$ (number of alternatives compared)

$= \log_2 (7)$ {i.e., columns 3 through 9}

$= 3$ {the nearest integer to $\log_2 (7)$, since $2^3 = 8$}.

The positive values of S(2), S(3), and S(4) yield the designation 1 1 1 1 1 1 1 for columns 3 through 9. Multiplying respectively S(9), S(10), S(12) to the compound statement S(2) · S(3) · S(4) gives

Conditions	Result						
	3	*4*	*5*	*6*	*7*	*8*	*9*
S(2) · S(3) · S(4) · S(9)	1	1	1	0	1	0	0
S(2) · S(3) · S(4) · S(10)	1	1	0	1	0	0	0
S(2) · S(3) · S(4) · S(12)	1	0	1	1	0	0	1

Table 2.2
Symptom-Diagnosis Complex with Ranked Search

		1	2	3	4	5	6	7	8	9	10	11	12	13	14	15	16
History:	S(1)	1	1	1	1	1	1	1	1	1	1	1	1	1	1	1	1
	S(2)	1	1	1	1	1	1	1	1	1	1	1	1	1	0	0	0
	S(3)	1	1	1	1	1	1	1	1	1	1	1	0	0	1	1	0
Physical Exam:	S(4)	1	1	1	1	1	1	1	1	1	0	0	0	1	1	0	0
	S(5)	1	1	0	0	0	0	0	0	0	1	1	1	0	0	0	0
	S(6)	1	1	0	0	0	0	0	0	0	0	0	0	1	1	1	1
Blood Tests:	S(7)	1	1	1	1	1	1	0	1	0	1	1	1	1	1	1	0
	S(8)	1	1	1	1	1	1	1	0	1	1	1	0	0	0	0	1
	S(9)	1	1	1	1	1	0	1	0	0	1	0	1	1	0	0	1
	S(10)	1	1	1	0	0	1	0	0	0	0	0	0	0	1	0	0
	S(11)	1	1	1	0	0	0	0	0	1	0	0	0	1	0	0	0
	S(12)	1	0	1	1	1	1	0	0	1	1	0	0	0	0	0	1
Marrow Tests:	S(13)	1	1	0	0	0	0	0	0	0	1	1	1	0	0	0	0
	S(14)	0	0	0	0	1	1	1	0	0	0	0	0	1	1	1	1
	D(1)	0	1	0	0	0	0	0	0	1	0	0	0	0	0	0	0
	D(2)	0	0	1	0	0	0	0	0	0	0	0	0	0	0	1	0
	D(3)	0	0	0	1	0	1	0	0	0	0	0	1	1	0	0	0
	D(4)	0	0	0	0	1	0	0	0	0	0	0	0	0	1	0	0
	D(5)	0	0	0	0	1	0	0	0	0	0	0	0	0	0	0	1
	D(6)	0	0	0	0	0	1	0	0	0	1	1	1	0	0	0	0
	D(7)	1	0	0	0	0	0	1	0	0	0	1	1	0	0	0	0
	D(8)	0	0	0	0	0	0	0	1	0	0	0	0	0	0	1	0

which are the same designations as the individual S(9), S(10), and S(12). Forming the compound statement S(9) · $\overline{S(10)}$ · S(12) reduces the columns 3 through 9 to the designation 0 0 1 0 0 0 0. This number is the one shown for D(4) and D(5) in Table 2.2. In summary, the positive history symptoms S(2) and S(3), when combined with the positive physical finding S(4), gave values of 1 in columns 3 through 9. Laboratory tests S(9), S(10), and S(12) were unaltered when combined (multiplicatively) with these history and physical conditions. The combination of laboratory results which reduces the product to a single positive finding was S(9) · $\overline{S(10)}$ · S(12). This result was in agreement with either diagnosis D(4) or D(5).

Table 2.3
Symptom-Diagnosis Complex Table

	1	2	3	4	5	6	7	8	9	10	11	12	13	14	15	16
A. History																
S(1)	1	1	1	1	1	1	1	1	1	1	1	1	1	1	1	1
S(2)	1	1	1	1	1	1	1	1	1	1	1	1	1	0	0	0
S(3)	1	1	1	1	1	1	1	1	1	1	1	0	0	1	1	0
S(1)·S(2)	1	1	1	1	1	1	1	1	1	1	1	1	1	0	0	0
S(1)·S(3)	1	1	1	1	1	1	1	1	1	1	1	1	0	1	1	0
S(2)·S(3)	1	1	1	1	1	1	1	1	1	1	1	0	0	0	0	0
B. Physical Exam																
S(4)	1	1	1	1	1	1	1	1	1	0	0					
S(5)	1	1	0	0	0	0	0	0	0	1	1					
S(6)	1	1	0	0	0	0	0	0	0	0	0					
S(4)·S(5)	1	1	0	0	0	0	0	0	0	0	0					
S(4)·S(6)	1	1	0	0	0	0	0	0	0	0	0					
S(5)·S(6)	1	1	0	0	0	0	0	0	0	0	0					
S(4)·$\overline{S(5)}$	0	0	1	1	1	1	1	1	1	0	0					
S(4)·$\overline{S(6)}$	0	0	1	1	1	1	1	1	1	0	0					
$\overline{S(5)}$·$\overline{S(6)}$	0	0	1	1	1	1	1	1	1	0	0					
C. Blood Tests																
S(7)			1	1	1	1	0	1	0							
S(8)			1	1	1	1	1	0	1							
S(9)			1	1	1	0	1	0	0							
S(10)			1	1	0	1	0	0	0							
S(11)			1	0	0	0	0	0	1							
S(12)			1	0	1	1	0	0	1							

Probability Tables

The logical diagnostic sequence may not come to a unique conclusion, and cost or feasibility factors may require an additional decision-making process. Consult Table 2.1, which illustrates probability table construction. According to that table, a patient had both symptoms S(1) and S(2) and symptom complexes 8, 12, and 16. A historical record of case histories showing the relationship between symptom complexes and diagnostic complexes is presented in Table 2.4.

Dividing each entry in Table 2.4 by 2,400, the total number of cases, yields the observed probabilities based on the historical data. These are

Table 2.4
Relationship Between Symptom Complex and Diagnosis Complex

		Symptom Complex				
		s^1	s^2	s^3	s^4	Total
Diagnosis Complex	d_1	0	0	0	0	
	d_2	0	600	300	300	1200
	d_3	0	0	300	300	600
	d_4	0	0	400	200	600
	Total	0	600	1000	800	2400

given in Table 2.5. The probabilities expressed in the row totals represent the relative frequencies of given diagnostic complexes ($P(d_j)$). The probabilities given in the column totals represent the frequency of observing the given symptom complexes ($P(s^i)$). Both probabilities ($P(d_j)$) and $P(s^i)$ are called *marginal probabilities.*

Conditional probability distributions are shown in Table 2.6. $P(s^i|d_j)$ is the probability of a particular symptom complex, given a diagnosis complex (Table 2.6, part A); $P(d_j|s^i)$ is the probability of a particular diagnosis complex, given a symptom complex (Table 2.6, part B).

Consider the patient with S(1) *and* S(2), which corresponds to the set of complexes cited in column 4 of Table 2.6B. The $P(d_1|s^4) = 0$; $P(d_2|s^4) = 3/8$; $P(d_3|s^4) = 3/8$; and $P(d_4|s^4) = 2/8$. These probabilities suggest that $d_2(D(1) \cdot \overline{D(2)})$ and $d_3(\overline{D(1)} \cdot D(2))$ occur with equal frequency and that $d_4(\overline{D(1)} \cdot D(2))$ occurs less frequently. These probabilities could be calculated using *Bayes' Formula:*

$$P(d_4|s^4) = \frac{P(d_4) \, P(s^4|d_4)}{\sum_k P(d_k) \, P(s^k|d_k)}, \; k = 1, \ldots 4.$$

Table 2.5
Estimated Probability Distribution

		Symptom Complex s^i				Total $P(d_j)$
		1	2	3	4	
Diagnosis Complex d_j	1	0	0	0	0	
	2	0	$\frac{6}{24}$	$\frac{3}{24}$	$\frac{3}{24}$	$\frac{12}{24}$
	3	0	0	$\frac{3}{24}$	$\frac{3}{24}$	$\frac{6}{24}$
	4	0	0	$\frac{4}{24}$	$\frac{2}{24}$	$\frac{6}{24}$
	Total $P(s^i)$	0	$\frac{6}{24}$	$\frac{10}{24}$	$\frac{8}{24}$	$\frac{24}{24}$

Table 2.6
Conditional Probabilities Using Marginal Frequencies

A. $P(s^i|d_j)$

		s^i				
		1	**2**	**3**	**4**	**Total**
	1	0	0	0	0	0
d_j	**2**	0	6/12	3/12	3/12	12
	3	0	0	3/6	3/6	6
	4	0	0	4/6	2/6	6
	$P(s^i)$		6/24	10/24	8/24	24

B. $P(d_j|s^i)$

		s^i				
		1	**2**	**3**	**4**	$P(d_j)$
	1	0	0	0	0	
d_j	**2**	0	6/6	3/10	3/8	12/24
	3	0	0	3/10	3/8	6/24
	4	0	0	4/10	2/8	6/24
	Total	0	6	10	8	24

Similarly, conditional probabilities for a particular symptom complex with a given diagnosis complex are

$$P(s^i|d_j) = \frac{P(s^i)\,P(d_j|s^i)}{\sum_k P(s^k)\,P(d_j|s^k)}$$

The *Bayes' Formula* makes it possible to translate from frequently provided data $P(s^i|d_j)$ to the required $P(d_j|s^i)$. Using Table 2.6, the numerator of the Bayes' Formula contains $P(d_j)$, that is, the probability that a given diagnostic complex will be observed, and is a characteristic of a given population at a given time; and $P(s^i|d_j)$, which is essentially independent of the current patient population and provides the structural knowledge of symptoms and diagnoses.

This Bayesian approach provides a mechanism for choosing among the alternative diagnoses by implying odds for each choice. These payoffs refer to the action taken as well as the diagnosis. As an example, consider the relationship in Table 2.7.

The pluses and minuses refer to the potential benefits of surgery. The safe strategy is to assume the patient has appendicitis. If the patient has mesenteric adenitis, not appendicitis, the disadvantage of surgery is a scar

Table 2.7
Diagnosis and Payoff

		Surgeon's Diagnosis	
		Acute Appendicitis	Mesenteric Adenitis
Patient has	Acute Appendicitis	+	−
	Mesenteric Adenitis	+	+

in the right iliac fossa. The danger of treating appendicitis as if it were mesenteric adenitis is prolonged illness. Strategies and payoffs will change as new diagnostics and therapeutics are introduced.

Decision Tree
Schwartz and co-workers illustrated the applications of decision analysis using the *decision tree* (1973). A decision tree consists of nodes and branches. There are two kinds of nodes. *Decision nodes* refer to those locations where the investigator chooses one action from amongst a presenting set of actions. *Chance nodes* designate responses from a course of action. These responses are described by conditional probability distributions (see Table 2.6). The decision tree scheme is shown in Figures 2.1 and 2.2.

The tree in Figure 2.1 depicts the flow of decisions and responses. The branches represent the courses stemming from a decision. The importance of the course of action is shown as a separate symbol in Figure 2.2. This graph more accurately depicts the process which involves at minimum

1. a decision influenced by the probabilities describing diagnosis and treatment potentials (the payoffs)
2. the courses of action and their risk/benefit considerations
3. the outcomes representing the conditional distributions given the course of action.

The graph in Figure 2.2, by calling attention to the courses as a separate entity, provides the opportunity to replace outmoded courses without modifying the basic structure.

The feasibility of working with the tree is enhanced by pruning unimportant branches. The intent is to construct a constrained tree representing the branches and nodes describing, in an optimal way, the problems in treating a particular patient. Trimming proceeds from the distal twigs and branches upward and inward. As with compound logical statements, branches can be collapsed to represent compound procedures. These would be expanded if needed later.

Fig. 2.1.
Decision Tree Format.

Decision --> Chance Relationship

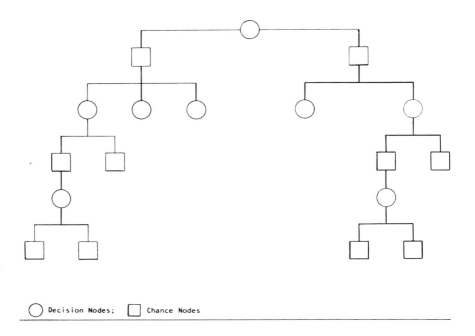

◯ Decision Nodes;   ☐ Chance Nodes

The quantification process involves three steps:

1. to estimate the probability of disease, given each test
2. to estimate the value judgments inherent in the course of action
3. to combine these factors for an expected value, allowing the various courses of action to be compared using the same scale.

There are two numerical estimates needed in order to invoke the Bayes' rule:

1. the *a priori* probability of the diagnosis based on clinical data
2. the accuracy of the procedure considered, that is, the frequency of false positive and false negative results

These estimates are in terms of previous notation (Table 2.6):

1. $P(d_j)$ = probability of diagnosis j in the population
2. $P(d_j|s^i)$ = probability of diagnosis j, given symptom i
3. $P(s^i|d_j)$ = probability of symptom i, given diagnosis j.

The latter probability set is most frequently maintained, and usually provides the false positive and false negative values.

Fig. 2.2.
Decision Tree Format.

```
Decision --> Course of Action --> Chance Relationship
```

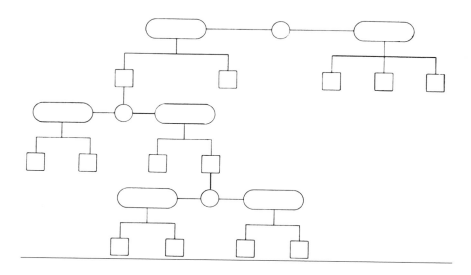

The example used by Schwartz (1973) involved a group of 1,000 hypertensive patients. The specific diagnosis in 950 patients was essential hypertension (EH) and, in the other 50, it was functional renal artery stenosis (FRAS). Suppose that 2% of the EH patients yielded positive results on renal arteriography and renal venous renins and 10% of the FRAS patients had negative findings with these studies. In this group of 1,000 patients, 19 with EH and 45 with FRAS would have positive studies. The probability that an individual with a positive test came from the FRAS group would be

$$P(A|S^+) = \frac{45}{45 + 19} = 0.70.$$

where

A   = functional renal artery stenosis
B   = essential hypertension
S^+ = positive studies.

The chance that the positive test came from the EH group would be

$$P(B|S^+) = \frac{19}{45 + 19} = 0.30.$$

Using the Bayes rule:

$$P(A|S^+) = \frac{P(A)P(S^+|A)}{P(A)P(S^+|A) + P(B) \cdot P(S^+|B)}$$

$$= \frac{(50/1000)(45/50)}{(50/1000)(45/50) + (950/1000) \cdot (19/950)}$$

$$= \frac{45/1000}{\dfrac{45}{1000} + \dfrac{19}{1000}}$$

$$= \frac{45}{45 + 19}$$

$$= 0.70.$$

In a similar fashion to false positive and false negative diagnostic results, the adverse and beneficial results from a specific therapy can be quantified.

With these probabilities identified, outcomes can be estimated. As an example, suppose that the tree were as shown in Figure 2.3. We assume

Fig. 2.3.
Probability Estimates.

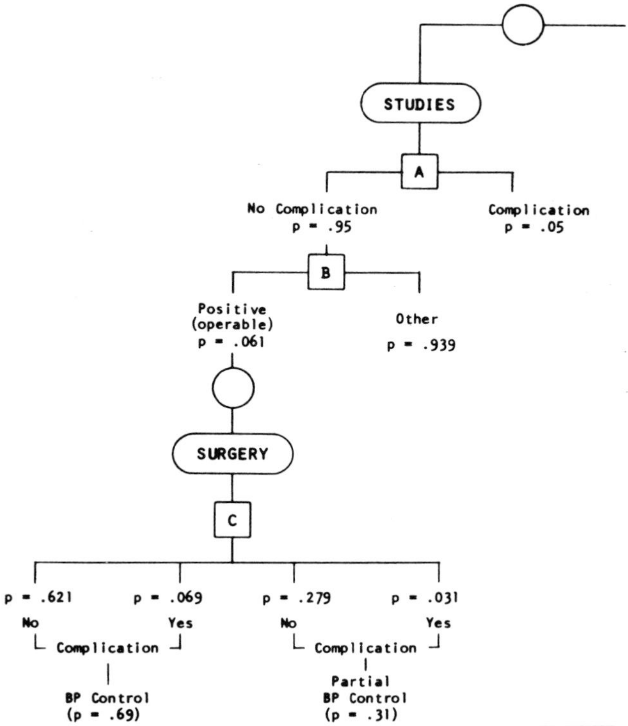

that the probability of complication from doing the study is 0.05. The probability of a favorable outcome, if surgery were performed, is 0.99. The formula stating this is

$$P(\text{Control}|\text{Pos OP}) = P(\text{Control}|\text{FRAS OP}) \cdot P(\text{FRAS OP}|\text{Pos OP}).$$

Therefore, the probability of blood pressure control, given a positive study result recommending surgery, is the product of:

1. probability of control, given the FRAS surgical procedure
2. probability of performing the surgery, given the positive study.

We can assume that

$$P(\text{FRAS OP}|\text{Pos OP}) = P(\text{FRAS}|\text{Pos}),$$

namely, that the FRAS is present, given a positive finding. This probability is 0.70. The probability of blood pressure control, given a positive study, then is

$$
\begin{aligned}
P(\text{Control}|\text{Pos OP}) &= P(\text{Control}|\text{FRAS OP}) \cdot P(\text{FRAS}|\text{Pos}) \\
&= (0.99)(0.70) \\
&= 0.69.
\end{aligned}
$$

Assuming a surgical complication occurred in 10% of cases:

$$
\begin{aligned}
P(&\text{Control with complication from surgery}) \\
&= P(\text{Control}|\text{Pos OP})P(\text{surgical complication}) \\
&= (0.69)(0.10) \\
&= 0.069.
\end{aligned}
$$

The probabilities of positive results, with surgery (chance node B in Figure 2.3), can be estimated by calculating the probability of a positive result in both the FRAS group and the EH group.

The positive (operative) finding may be estimated by:

$$
\begin{aligned}
P(\text{Pos}|\text{FRAS}) + P(\text{Pos}|\text{EH}) &= 0.90 + 0.02 \\
&= 0.92.
\end{aligned}
$$

The positive finding group thus makes up 0.92 (proportion "called" FRAS), which gives 0.92 (0.05 + 0.02) = .0644. As shown in Figure 2.3, 95% of these have positive findings without complications from the studies, or 0.0644 (0.95) = 0.061. Approximately 0.94% of those without complications will have other than positive findings.

The value (worth, importance, desirability) of each outcome may be transformed by the investigator into numerical expressions of his feelings about the outcomes. For the purposes of the present example using Figure 2.3, assume that the four final outcomes were given the "worths":

1. blood pressure control   no complications   50
                                  complications -40

2. partial control   no complications -25
                                  complications -50

These numbers suggest:

1. The best result ($+50$) is control without complications.
2. Partial control without complications, given a value of (-25), implies that this result is far less desirable than the best.
3. Control with complications (-40) is only slightly better than
4. Partial control with complications (-50).

The size of these numbers must satisfy the following conditions:

Ranked Choices	Size	Condition
1	S_1	$S_1 > S_2 + S_3 + S_4$
2	S_2	$S_2 > S_3 + S_4$
3	S_3	$S_3 > S_4$
4	S_4	

The *expected value* of a chance node with a p_1 chance of consequence 1, p_2 chance of 2, . . . is

$$EV = p_1V_1 + p_2V_2 + \ldots + p_nV_n$$

where there are n possibilities with values $V_1, V_2, \ldots V_n$ and probabilities of occurrence, p_i, $i = 1, 2, \ldots n$.

The expected value of chance node C (Figure 2.3) is then:

$$
\begin{aligned}
EV_c &= (0.621)(50) + (0.069)(-40) + (0.279)(-25) + (0.031)(-50) \\
&= (31.05) + (-2.76) + (-6.975) + (-1.55) \\
&= 19.765.
\end{aligned}
$$

At chance node B, there are two outcomes, the positive-operable leading to node C with value 19.765 and probability 0.062, and the other with probability 0.938. Assume that the value associated with the latter outcome is -20. This branch represents partial control without surgery. The expected value of node B is

$$
\begin{aligned}
EV_B &= 0.061(19.765) + 0.939(-20) \\
&= 1.20566 + (-18.78) \\
&= -17.57.
\end{aligned}
$$

The expected value at node A is then

$$EV_A = (0.95)(-17.57) + (0.05)(-40)$$

where -40 represents the value of the branch associated with complications from the diagnostic studies and partial control without surgery

$$
\begin{aligned}
EV_A &= (-16.6915) + (-2) \\
&= -18.69.
\end{aligned}
$$

To summarize these findings and to re-iterate their use, the expected value of chance outcome A represents the results of performing the diagnostic studies associated with surgery. One would choose this path if EV_A were superior to its alternative. EV_B and EV_C represent the expected values for subsequent chance events along this path. EV_C is the expected value of surgery to control blood pressure with and without complications. EV_B is the expected value of surgical versus drug control when the positive versus other diagnostic findings are considered. The tree's complexity, the expected values at chance nodes, and their composition in terms of path values may be used to decide the appropriate course of action.

The values assigned and their reproducibility are areas of concern. The specific values assigned may be less important than their ranking and relative weights. For example:

  let A represent a favored outcome, and
    B, an unfavored one;

  let p represent the frequency of A, and
    $(1 - p)$, the frequency of B.

Now

  let C represent a third outcome.

Depending on the value of p, and the frequencies of A's and B's, a preference between C and the chance selection A versus B would choose A instead of C if p were close to 1. The preference would be C instead of B if p were close to 0. For some value of p, say p^1, there will be indifferences between the result C and the results of chance selection A versus B. This chance selection, A versus B, is called a lottery. The expected value of C would be

$$EV(C) = p^1 V(A) + (1 - p^1) V(B).$$

As shown in the calculations using the decision tree in Figure 2.3, the expected value associated with an outcome may be computed by using probabilities reflecting frequencies of the outcomes. These probabilities weight the worth assigned to each. In formal utility theory, the outcomes are assumed to be different in worth, so that the probability, p^1, could be chosen to represent no difference between the outcomes. The expected value calculations then are

$$EV\ (Event) = \sum_{i=1}^{k} (\text{probability of occurrence})\ (\text{Worth})$$

or

$$EV\ (Event) = p^1\ Value\ I + (1 - p^1)\ Value\ II$$

where p^1 is a proportion between 0 and 1 representing that point at which Value I and Value II are equal in preference. At that point, Event may be equal in preference to the lottery involving events I and II.

Summary
The basic structure used in clinical decision analysis is the hierarchical graph depicting the sequence of alternatives involved in the diagnosis and treatment process. The graph can be used for making decisions if there are data to supply the required numerical values. The key data needed are

1. probability distributions representing outcomes
2. beneficial and adverse effects of treatment
3. duration of illness and survival results which are relevant to outcome.

Chapter 3

Historical and Current Guidelines for Medical Trials

Introduction
There have been a number of articles dealing with the medical trial, several of which have been selected for presentation in this chapter, which discusses guidelines for planning and conducting research. The time period represented by these examples, 1958 to 1977, is relatively short; however, that period in history witnessed an enormous outpouring of funds and effort directed to the study and solution of health problems.

Notes on Planning and Evaluation of Research
A three part series in the American Heart Journal in 1958 dealt with this topic (Mainland 1958). The problem leading to these discussions was, in the author's view, as follows:

To those of us who engage in medical research, it often seems as if Nature were laying traps on every hand, to prevent our reaching the truth. Unfortunately, many of us discover these traps only when the product of months of painstaking work is refused publication because inadequate planning has led to ill-founded conclusions.

In an attempt to suggest guidelines to reduce this *wasted effort,* Dr. Mainland posed ten sets of questions:

With change of tense from future to past, this series of questions becomes a scheme for the basic "statistical" evaluation of a report on work already done. This is more fundamental than arithmetical tests; without it, the arithmetic is meaningless and dangerous.

The first questions dealt with purpose and basic structure. These were

I-1. What is the immediate purpose of our investigation? That is, what are the specific questions to be answered by it?

I-2. What is the more remote (more general or ultimate) purpose of our investigation?

I-3. Will the investigation be an experiment, in the strict sense?—A Survey?—Both?

I-4. If the investigation is a survey, will it be anecdotal or statistical?

I-5. If the investigation is a survey, will it be retrospective or prospective?

I-6. If the investigation is a survey, is there a hypothetical experiment which, if it were possible, we would perform instead of the survey?

These questions focus the planner's attention to the first of a series of branching paths (Figure 3.1) depicting the *design process.* This first step involves the selection of a specific immediate purpose to be accomplished by the study. This goal should reflect a general concept and thus a basic design. As seen in Figure 3.1, there are two forms: the experiment and the survey.

Fig. 3.1.
Initial Branches in Research Design Planning.

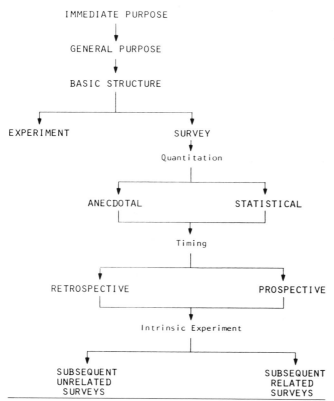

The experiment, Mainland considered, satisfied two characteristics:

1. The individuals being studied received the element to be tested by a device independent of the individuals.
2. The assignment of test element was performed in a fashion which eliminated or minimized known sources of bias.

The survey then satisfied neither of these conditions. In the survey, the element considered (not tested) was an attribute of the individual studied (and thus dependent upon him). Further, the assignment of attribute to individual was not performed by a known method. Indeed, the purpose of the survey could be associated with "discovering" the conditions and features describing the assignment process.

Mainland, in differentiating between experiment and survey, offered the following example:

The amount of interference with, or manipulation of, our test material is not a criterion of experimentation. For example, an investigator wished to compare intravascular blood pressures in cardiac and noncardiac diseases. He inserted needles into the brachial arteries, catheters into the pulmonary arteries, and needles into the jugular bulbs. Since he had not assigned the factors under test (cardiac and noncardiac disease) to the subjects, he conducted a survey, just as if he had compared male and female statures.

The second series of questions referred to the sampling process and, in particular, the sample space. These questions were

II-1. What is the initial definition of our population or universe, i.e., the kind of subjects or material to be studied, and to which our conclusions will be applicable?

II-2. What other populations are excluded by the definition given in response to Question II-1?

II-3. If all the available subjects of our chosen population are not to be investigated, how is the sample to be taken?

II-4. If the sample is not to be taken by a strictly automatic random process, how may the sampling method affect the definition of the population?

The intent of these questions is to characterize, in word form, the necessary attributes possessed by each individual to be studied. Those individuals lacking one or more of the attribute set would be excluded. The population or universe of individuals with the required set is ascertained by appropriate answers to relevant questions. All other individuals constitute a second population or universe, because they are not members of the chosen first set. This is illustrated in Figures 3.2 and 3.3.

Fig. 3.2.
Definition of Population.

Exclusive Attributes

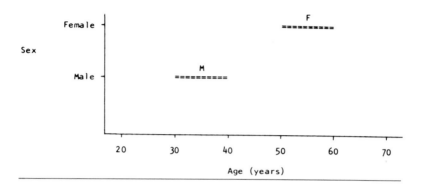

In Figure 3.2, the individuals may be characterized by the two variates, age and sex. As seen, the males and females were grouped separately by age. In Figure 3.3, the age difference remains constant between the two sexes. The systolic blood pressure values were different for each sex, but some values were common to both.

Fig. 3.3.
Definition of Population.

Shared Attributes

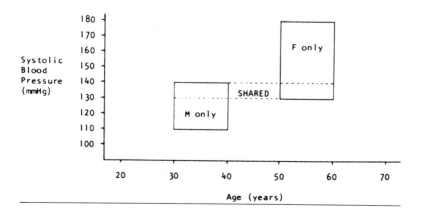

Fig. 3.4.
Selection of Individuals from a Population.

Non-Random Selection Rule

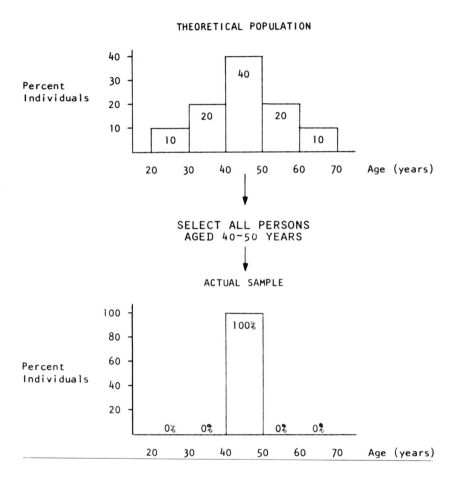

THEORETICAL POPULATION

SELECT ALL PERSONS
AGED 40-50 YEARS

ACTUAL SAMPLE

In Figure 3.2, either age or sex could distinguish the groups. However, blood pressure results overlap and make separation by sex or age impossible (Figure 3.3). Therefore, selection of unique subgroups no longer is possible.

The second concern posed by these questions is the capacity of the study to include all of the appropriate persons. Indeed, this concern is more theoretical than real, in that it is never possible. The population, as defined, is larger than the number of available individuals, so that the latter must represent a *sample* of the population. The methods used to obtain individuals for membership in the sample group is critical. Mainland's last question focuses on the difficulties in interpretation which exist when the available sample does not accurately represent the entire population. This requirement of "strict representation" can be accomplished only through the use of random selection. This allows each individual in the population to have the same chance of being included in the sample. Further, each individual is independent in the selection process. This phenomenon is illustrated in Figures 3.4 and 3.5.

Nonrandom selection procedures are shown in Figure 3.4. The upper part of the figure is a frequency distribution representing the population of interest. With a nonrandom rule, the sample selected could be grossly nonrepresentative of the population. In contrast, with random selection,

Fig. 3.5.
Selection of Individuals from a Population.

Random Selection Rule

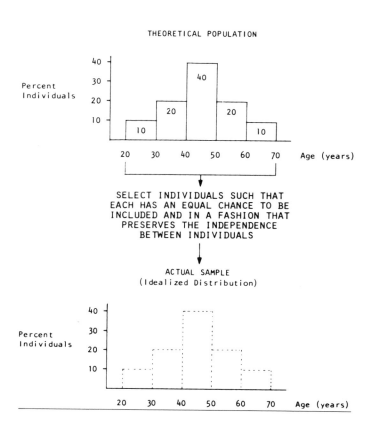

THEORETICAL POPULATION

Percent Individuals

SELECT INDIVIDUALS SUCH THAT
EACH HAS AN EQUAL CHANCE TO BE
INCLUDED AND IN A FASHION THAT
PRESERVES THE INDEPENDENCE
BETWEEN INDIVIDUALS

ACTUAL SAMPLE
(Idealized Distribution)

Percent Individuals

the expected sample distribution would more closely approximate the theoretical one (Fig. 3.5).

The third question set was intended to facilitate understanding of the difficulties in relating population attributes, samples representing the population, and interpretations of the study findings. The questions were

III-1. *Why do we subdivide (stratify or systematically subsample) our population and test the factors under Study (A, B, etc.) within each subsample or stratum?*

III-2. *What, in the form of a list, are the factors (in addition to the factors under test) that affect, or could conceivably affect, the phenomena to be observed?*

III-3. *Which of the factors listed in answer to Question III-2 are to be used in subdivision of the population?*

III-4. *Why are the other factors listed in answer to Question III-2 not to be used in subdivision of the population?*

III-5. *Why are the subdivisions of the population not to be coarser or finer?*

III-6. *Are we going to make paired comparisons, i.e., within the same subject, or between subjects that are matched in some way? If so, why?*

These questions were developed to illustrate a number of issues. Stratification of a population and subsequent selection of samples from each stratum are important procedures in accomplishing the following objectives:

1. Reduction of Misclassification (Mislabeling)
   The labeling of an attribute or of a phenomenon is an automatic behavior. In science, this automatic behavior becomes a conscious one, and the identification methods and the criteria for group assignment become the province of the scientific discipline. The attention to subpopulations implied in Question III-1 attempts to reinforce the importance of class definition and reduce the error of mislabeling. If this error is reduced in size and impact, the likelihood is increased that findings will be appropriately interpreted.

2. Reduction of Variation
   In addition to initial mislabeling, there is the problem of mislabeling associated with outcome. This is observed most frequently in terms of treatment. The misrecognition is illustrated in Figure 3.6. Two treatments, new and old, are compared in presumably one type of disease. Actually, two groups of patients are included; both long survival, and short survival. These two groups, when combined, show survival ranging from small to large. This variation is due exclusively to the mixing of patients. As seen in Figure 3.6, when patients

Fig. 3.6.
Mislabeling and Varying Subclass Behavior.

A. Mislabeling Two Groups as One

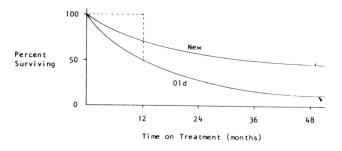

B. Stratified Samples

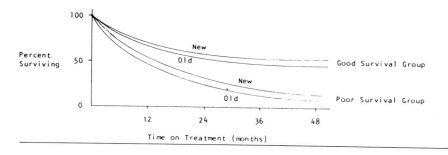

are mislabeled as one disease and assigned to treatment, an assignment, even random, could allot the new agent to more long-term survivors. The consequence would be a significantly longer survival in the group receiving NEW as compared to those receiving OLD, and the treatment would be mistakenly considered as the reason for the longevity. If the inherent survival potential were recognized in the assignment process and random assignment to treatment performed within these strata, the figure would show that there was no difference between OLD and NEW treatments. In Figure 3.6, part B, there is no mislabeling associated with treatment. Indeed, there is no mislabeling of the groups in terms of initial or subsequent factors.

The questions concerning the identification (in the form of a list) of pertinent factors, which could be used to define subgroups, and the reduction of that list to those factors actually used had for their object the motivation of a rationale, a justification for the sampling design. Inherent in this exercise is the reliance on previous knowledge (e.g., literature, past work, etc.) to assist in the definition. Two concepts are considered:

1. The new research should build upon, improve, and expand the foundations of accepted knowledge.

2. That foundation should be defined in the most precise terms, in order to accurately sample and to insure appropriate extrapolations from the sampling results.

An operational issue is the ease in reproducing the results. The stratification rules should be made explicit so that they can be applied by others intending to replicate the study design and test the findings.

Question III-6 represents an important design element. It involves the use of the individual in recognition of a change with time, treatment, or other influence, and the selection of two individuals presumably identical to each other for development of a measure of difference. The first process, a standard format, includes multiple measures of the same individual through time. The resulting data may be a series of time-linked records or a single datum representing the change with time. A number of analytical models have been developed for the latter situation. The analysis of series of time-linked records represents a more recent effort.

The pairing or matching design has appealed to scientists studying characteristics in litters of animals. The assumption of minimal difference and variation is satisfied more readily in genetically pure strains. This assumption fails in human research. Matching criteria thus became important in assessing the information potential.

The fourth set of questions deals with display and analysis of potential results. The questions were

IV-1. How, in skeleton form, will the results appear?

IV-2. Are measurements to be presented as (a) mensuration data (e.g., as means or variations), or as (b) enumeration data (e.g., in contingency tables)? What will determine the choice between (a) and (b)?

IV-3. What do we expect to be the order of magnitude of the frequencies and measurements—e.g., percentage of X's in A's, means of measurements, variations between measurements?

IV-4. Are the sampling units correct?

IV-5. Are the denominators correct?

IV-6. How may the structure of our measurements mislead us?

The precise analysis to be used is an important component in the information potential of the study. The first question refers to the form chosen to

Fig. 3.7.
Summary of Elements Relating Research Processes with Purpose.

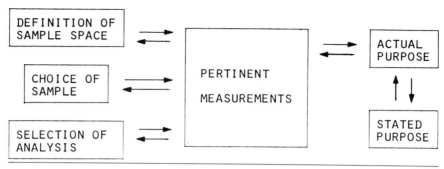

illustrate the relationship between the purpose of the study and the display of results. This connection involves the other relationships described by the previous question sets, which are summarized in Figure 3.7. The interactions between the *sampling space,* the *sample* chosen, and the *analytical plan* relate to the measurements used. These, in turn, shape the actual purpose. A successful design would have a close agreement between the intended or stated purpose and the actual one.

Questions IV-2 and IV-3 apply to the selection of the best descriptive term for a concept or attribute. While selection may be determined by the form of analysis to be used, it also is influenced by existing practice. Description of a group in terms of mensuration data would include such numerical values as the mean, standard deviation, or range. For example, the group could be described using age by

1. mean = 20 years
2. standard deviation = 5 years
3. range = 15–30 years.

This same group could be described using concepts of enumeration by choosing the interval 15 to 30 to represent those who would be labeled as "young." In the former, the actual ages play an essential role in the description. In the latter, the actual ages are irrelevant once the value has been judged to be within the critical interval. This suppression of information may be viewed as a mechanism for reducing "noise." The mensuration approach may be viewed as precise, because of the influence of each datum. The investigator must then choose the approach, using the criterion of maximum information potential to the problem rather than a standard format.

Having selected the form of presentation, whether it is to be mensuration or enumeration, the analytical structure can be expected to yield information desired within the limits of the intended sampling. That is, given the analytical model, the size of the sample required to obtain interpretable results should be considered. The sample size illustrates the need for compromise between performance costs and information derived. The likelihood of satisfying the study purpose is related closely to the measurements, their distribution in the various subgroups studied, and the analysis chosen to demonstrate these facts. The lack of precise knowledge at the time of planning should motivate careful consideration of the validity of results obtained under these conditions. Sample sizes should be chosen to protect against such waste within the constraints of costs, effort, and facilities.

Question IV-4 illustrates a continuing need to assess agreement between assumptions and conditions of the analytical model and the individuals and data to be obtained. If the model does not describe the real situation, the analytical results cannot.

The question of choosing the correct denominator deals with mislabeling problems. Choice of individuals to compose an appropriate analytical group may be difficult, since individuals may possess multiple characteristics, and analysis frequently can focus on only one or two. This is illustrated in Figure 3.8, which depicts individuals defined first by age and sex. They are then assigned treatment. The final results are shown last.

Comparison of the displays (Figures 3.8 and 3.9) indicates the potential problems in selecting appropriate subgroups. In Figure 3.8, the total number of persons is separated into subgroups using the sequence of variates and criteria:

1. age
2. sex
3. treatment
4. outcome.

In Figure 3.9, the sequence is

1. treatment
2. sex
3. age
4. outcome.

Since a particular subgroup exists in both distributions, choice of the total group used to calculate occurrence of outcomes may be "logically" valid or invalid, depending upon intent and perspective. The danger lies in using distributions such as that shown in Figure 3.9. The logical error is in categorizing the distribution by treatment and then identifying the *a priori* characteristics in the treatment groups. This behavior is appropriate when the characteristics may be assigned and not when they are observed.

The structure of measurements (Question IV-6) introduces a series of issues which will be considered in more detail subsequently. The important

Fig. 3.8.
Identification of Pertinent Groups in Analysis.

Group Definition using Pre-Treatment Characteristics

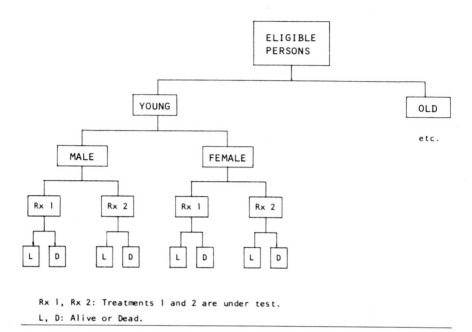

Rx 1, Rx 2: Treatments 1 and 2 are under test.
L, D: Alive or Dead.

preliminary concern in planning is redundancy in measurement. Two forms
of redundancy are common:

1. Duplication of data capture using different instruments, as happens
    when a patient is asked to provide his age, date of birth, date of
    marriage, and similar time variates reflecting age. This redundancy
    may be unimportant in deciding the individual's correct age. As multi-
    ple predictors of some outcome, however, the variates either intro-
    duce random error or hamper ability to identify the important age-
    related variate if it exists.

2. Variates purportedly representing separate components of dependent
    functions. For example, use A to predict R, where R is made of
    A + B. A will always be related to A. The strength of the relationship
    between A and (A + B) will depend on B. The "masking" of A by
    R (as A + B) is a device used in describing physiological functions.
    Care must be taken to insure that the description is real, not an
    artifact.

Fig. 3.9.
Identification of Pertinent Groups in Analysis.

Group Definition using Treatment Assignment

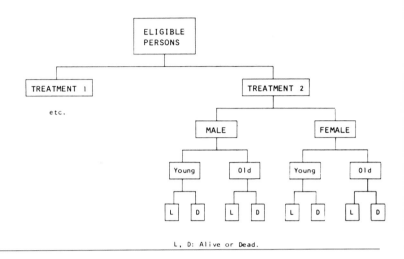

L, D: Alive or Dead.

The fifth set of questions deals with the problems of interpreting results from the anticipated study. The questions posed by Mainland were

V-1. *How shall we decide whether the results prove, or fail to prove, that the factors under test were responsible for the differences in outcome in the samples that were compared—(a) By inspection of the results in the light of our previous experience (e.g., experience of observational error, average level, and variability of animal responses)? (b) By a formal test of "statistical significance"?*

V-2. *If method (a) is to be used, what specifically (numerically) is the experience or background knowledge?*

V-3. *If method (b)—a formal test of "significance"—is proposed, and the investigation is an experiment, what precautions will be taken in order to make possible an inference of the form "either chance or the factors under test"?*

V-4. *If the investigation is a survey, or an experiment not conducted along the lines indicated under Question V-3, what would a test of "significance" tell us? Would it be helpful?*

V-5. *If a significance test is to be applied, what does it mean in terms of an experiment conducted with chance? What assumptions underlie the test? What is the evidence that they are valid for our data?*

V-6.   If a "significance" test is to be applied, what level of significance
       will be adopted as the critical level? Why was it chosen?

V-7.   What are the various possible outcomes of the investigation? What
       would be our action—our next step—in each case?

V-8.   How shall we estimate what our results really tell us, numerically,
       about the population represented by our samples?

V-9.   Do we intend, after the investigation, to search in the data for factors,
       effects, or relationships other than those that we contemplated when
       we designed the investigation? If so, how shall we interpret the find-
       ings? What risks do we run?

These questions emphasize major areas of concern within the context
of interpretation. These are

1.   The choice of an analytical model transcends computational feasibil-
     ity. The search is for the "truth" as expressed through the experi-
     ence of the study subjects. While the issue of subjective interference
     in analysis is clear in questions V-1 through V-3, the critical concern
     is matching the analytical structure with reality.
2.   The conduct of the study becomes relevant when interpretation of
     results is at hand. The methods of managing the subjects can con-
     tribute to identifying sources of error. Mainland emphasizes this by
     the phrase—"an inference of the form 'either chance or the factors
     under test.'" The two alternatives can be expanded to (1) *chance,*
     which implies that *only* measurement and procedural errors influ-
     enced the outcome; (2) *study factors,* which implies that *only* the
     variates and procedures described in the design influenced the out-
     come; and (3) *extraneous factors,* which implies that *only* variates
     and procedures omitted from consideration influenced the outcome.

The latter is an error of important magnitude, in that it implies the design
ignored relevant issues and concepts. If we assume that the studied factors
alone influenced the outcome, there is a choice of statistical methods to
perform the translations. If chance or extraneous factors were operating,
then these statistical procedures would not be helpful.

The remaining question sets deal with operational problems. The sixth set
was

VI-1.   If the investigation is a survey, how will the samples for comparison
        (A, B, etc.) be selected?

VI-2.   If the investigation is a survey, what will be the known or conceiv-
        able differences between the samples labeled "A," "B," etc., in
        addition to the factors or features that these letters represent?

VI-3. Will the selection of samples for comparison be in any way affected by the contents of the samples, i.e., by the percentage frequencies or measurements that they contain?

VI-4. How shall we decide when to stop the investigation?

The problems in selection have been touched on previously. Inclusion-exclusion criteria, with mechanisms for assessing compliance, will be discussed in greater detail subsequently.

The seventh question set presented by Mainland included

VII-1. What could conceivably make the selection rates of A, B, etc., differ from each other?
(Note that A, B are designators for groups.)

VII-2. What could conceivably make the selection rates of X and not-X (or X, Y, Z, etc.) differ from each other?
(Note that X, Y, Z are attributes.)

VII-3. Is there any assurance that competition between selection rates will not lead to Berkson's fallacy?
NOTE: If our answer to this question is based on assumptions, we must state them explicitly.

VII-4. Visualizing the period before we make the survey, is it conceivable that a phenomenon under study (X, not-X) will eliminate some subjects, by death or other means, and so prevent our including them in the surveys? If so, is it conceivable that this effect will differ in degree in As and Bs? That is, may prevalence mislead us regarding incidence (Neyman's fallacy)?

VII-5. If, in spite of the risks of bias from selection rates, and other inevitable uncertainties in surveys (Question V-4), we intend to conduct a survey, what is our justification for doing so?

Mainland's last question in this set suggests that he felt the dangers in misinterpretation of surveys far exceeded the benefits. While there is support for his conclusion, the survey can *generate new ideas.* Differences in inclusion of subgroups and consequently in outcomes (Berkson's fallacy) can occur and inappropriate comparisons of incidence and prevalence (Neyman's fallacy) can be made. These *mistakes in proving causality* are trivial in comparison with the opportunities to discover new relationships to test. Defects in the investigative process include errors in

1. defining and utilizing optimal sampling space
2. conducting the study
3. matching analysis with reality
4. providing correct interpretations.

Quantitative feasibility in the performance of the study is considered in the eighth set of questions. These were

VIII-1.   What sample sizes will be used in each group (A, B, etc.)?

VIII-2.   Will the samples be large enough to answer our questions?

VIII-3.   Will our facilities (personnel, time, money, etc.) suffice to produce the amount of information that we need?

Emphasis on quantity, while a necessary condition, is not the only consideration. This is evident when considering the management requirements necessary for one study subject. Can the design requirements be satisfied, given the limits of personnel, facilities, and funds for capturing the data, recording, storing, and analyzing these values? If not, increasing the sample size will only compound problems. If the process will work for one, will it work for two, three, . . . n subjects studied simultaneously? The sample size issue may be viewed in terms of:

1.   the number to be processed at one time, and
2.   the number of such groups required to provide the specified probability of recognizing the anticipated study outcome.

The next question set dealt with data collection. The questions were

IX-1.   Who?—Persons, i.e., observers, subjects, and others involved in the investigation.

IX-2.   What?—Events.

IX-3.   Where?—Location and environment.

IX-4.   When?—Time relationships.

IX-5.   How?—Methods.

IX-6.   When the possibility of bias is suggested by any of the preceding five questions, will the risk be (1) removed, e.g., by standardization of techniques, or (2) controlled by randomization?

The last set of questions was

X-1.   What can we confidently expect to be the percentage completeness of our samples at the beginning and throughout the investigation?

X-2.   How are we going to insure that the percentage completeness of our samples will be as high as possible?

X-3.   What numerical effects would the anticipated numbers of lost cases have on our conclusions?

X-4.   Will records be made of all subjects who, according to our plan, ought to have been in our samples, but who were omitted at the start or were lost later? Will the records give reasons for each omission?

X-5. *What will be the effects of missing items of data in past records, and of observations omitted during the investigation?*

X-6. *Do we expect to reject any observations? If so, on what grounds? Could these rejections introduce bias?*

Experimental Design of Clinical Trials
In 1973, Gehan and Schneiderman discussed the issues in human treatment research. The protocol, as described by them, was as follows:

. . . a written document outlining the purpose of the study including the rationale, the method of administering the treatments, and details concerning the plan of investigation. The elements of a protocol . . .

1. *Introduction and scientific background for the study*
2. *Objectives of study*
3. *Selection of patients*
4. *Design of study (including schematic diagram)*
5. *Treatment programs*
6. *Procedures in event of response, no response or toxicity*
7. *Required clinical and laboratory data*
8. *Criteria for evaluating the effect of treatment*
9. *Statistical considerations*
10. *Informed consent*
11. *Record forms*
12. *References*
13. *Study chairman or responsible investigator and telephone number.*

In addition to the structure of the protocol, Gehan and Schneiderman outlined the basic designs used in clinical trials. These were

1. Phase I Studies
Purpose—To determine a dosage regimen that is not too toxic and that can be used in looking for therapeutic effect.

2. Phase II Studies
Purpose—To determine whether a particular dosage schedule of an agent is active enough to warrant further study.

3. Follow-up Trial
Purpose—To provide estimate of effectiveness of an agent with specified precision.

4. Comparative Trial
Purpose—To decide whether new therapy is superior to standard therapy or not.

Fig. 3.10.
Additional Branches in Research Design Planning.

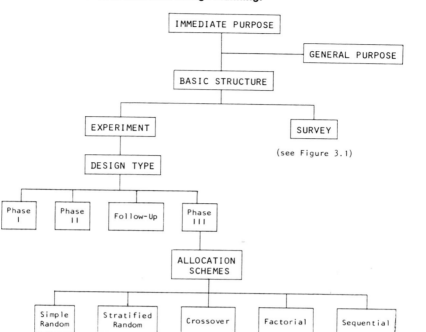

Expanding on the designs in the comparative trial type, Gehan and Schneiderman identified those shown in Figure 3.10. The *simple random* and *stratified* schemes have been discussed. The *crossover* scheme is a combination of a simple random design comparing two or more treatment regimens. The patient receives both regimens in random order. The typical flow is shown in Figure 3.11.

The *factorial* design tests the effects of multiple treatments, separately and in combination. The simplest of these factorial formats would be the "2 × 2" as shown in Figure 3.12. Note that the individual would be assigned randomly to one of the four groups.

Factorial designs may employ many treatments and dosage levels. For each cell subgroup of treatments and dosages considered, a certain minimum number of subjects is required. With ten to a cell, the 2 × 2 design would require 40 subjects. A 3 × 3 design would require 90. Some of the possible combinations may not be advisable to use, because known antagonisms within the set may have harmful effects. The emphasis on tolerable schedules would eliminate such combinations without study, thus fractionating the complete factorial structure. The use of fractional factorial designs is a more common practice in clinical trials.

Fig. 3.11.
Crossover Design Structure.

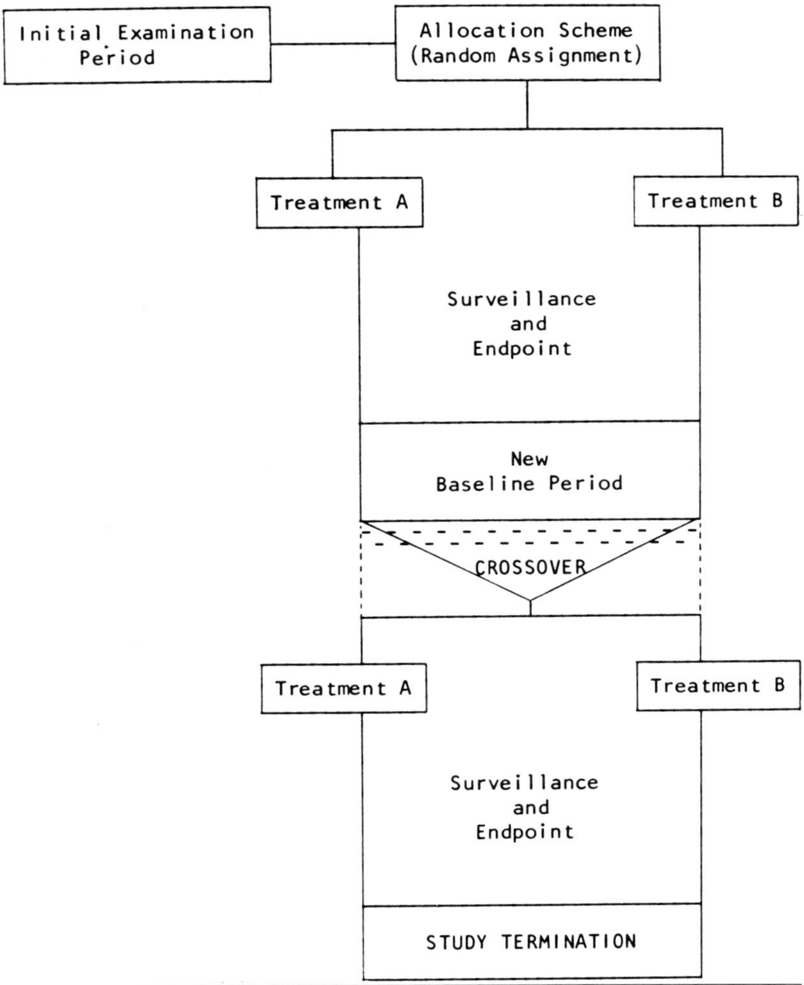

The *sequential* design offers the opportunity to perform repeated interim analyses without jeopardizing the final results as badly as in the fixed sample designs. The structure of the sequential trial is shown in Figure 3.13. Decision limits representing cessation of the trial were constructed prior to the onset of the study. Subjects are entered sequentially into the study and assigned the therapy at random. Each subject's outcome is plotted. The graph is structured so that agreement with the superiority of one therapy is a vertical movement. Agreement with the other therapy is a horizon-

Fig. 3.12.
Assignment to Treatment in 2 × 2 Factorial Design.

Flow Description

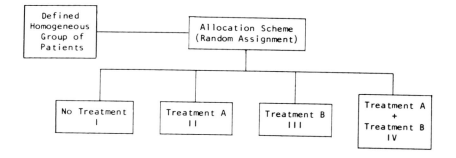

Usual Representation

tal movement. As long as the patient experience remains within defined boundaries, the study continues.

The study is terminated when a boundary is crossed or, in certain designs, when it is clear that "no decision" will be reached.

Design and Analysis of Randomized Clinical Trials
In December 1976 and January 1977, a report to the Medical Research Council's Leukemia Steering Committee was published in the *British Journal of Cancer* (Peto et al.). This report was prepared by statisticians from Britain and the United States. The intent of the report was to address *the more quantifiable aspects of clinical trials—treatment comparisons, treatment toxicities, treatment effects in special subgroups, recognition of*

Fig. 3.13.
Sequential Design Structure.

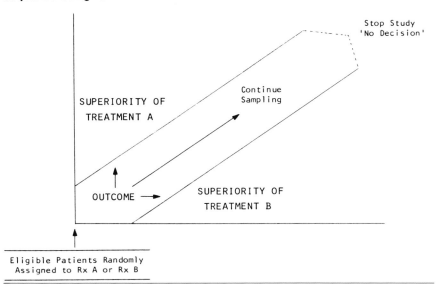

prognostic features, and so on—while ignoring the important indirect benefits of clinical trials.

The major statements in the report are given below:

1.   Whatever index of failure is of interest, one should not only count
     how many people "fail" but also see when they failed.

2.   Study of a few dozen patients can in most cases detect an ideal treat-
     ment which prevents more than two-thirds of the deaths, but more
     realistic effects, such as preventing about one-third of the deaths,
     requires well over 100 patients to be detected.

3.   A positive result is more likely, and a null result is more informative,
     if the main comparison is of only two treatments, these being as dif-
     ferent as possible.

4.   P = 0.05 does not mean "the probability that the treatments are
     equivalent is 0.05."

5.   A given P-value in a large trial is usually stronger evidence that the
     treatments really differ than the same P-value in a small trial of the
     same treatments would be.

6.   It is proper to combine prior opinion and knowledge with P-values
     to guess the truth.

7. What may be inferred if there is no statistically significant difference between two treatments?

8. Unequal allocation may be best.

9. Assessing a new treatment solely by comparison with past experience can be misleading; at least one-third of current patients should be randomized controls.

10. Balanced randomization at the latest possible time is recommended, with no stratification.

11. If, during analysis, initial prognosis will be allowed for while the different treatments are being compared, there is hardly ever need for stratification at entry in large trials.

12. Rigorous entry criteria are not necessary for a randomized trial, but rigorous follow-up is. Even patients who do not get the proper treatment must not be withdrawn from the analysis.

13. Early analysis of a trial can be misleading if a temporary difference, which would have been smoothed out by large numbers, causes the trial to be aborted so that large numbers never accumulate.

14. Individuals must never be denied clearly appropriate treatment, even if trial protocols are thereby disrupted.

These statements, with the associated explanations and discussion, may be summarized as follows:

1. A simple, comparative design with sufficient numbers of patients and a sensitive criterion of effect is best.

2. The complexities introduced by exceptions should be avoided.

3. These complexities may be dealt with effectively by analysis and the investigator must be prepared to understand "more difficult" analytical models when required by the problem.

4. The essence of the clinical trial begins and ends with dedicated, disciplined data capture and reporting. All patients eligible and entered must be followed. Later events must be subjected to analysis, in order to decide the relationships between entry factors, therapy, and outcome.

Protocol Development
As seen, these guidelines and conceptual structures assist the investigator in *thinking about* his research. Our experience suggests that this is insufficient. That is, methods are required to assist the investigators in *thinking through* their research. In most situations, the research is not simple. It may

well be a combination of both experiment and survey. Each study subject represents a detailed and dynamically evolving experience, beginning at entry with an assessment of prior events and findings, and concluding with the final evaluation and outcome. This patient management process is a major portion of the protocol, as it is considered by investigators in describing their research.

The second part, study management, is a detailed and dynamically evolving experience beginning with entry of the first study subjects and concluding with last report. This also is a process and, as such, is subject to alteration for the benefit or detriment of the study. This last idea was alluded to by the caution regarding early analysis and premature modification or cessation. Study management incorporates the essential aspects of patient and data management by formulating procedures and criteria for processing both. Analytical methods and decision criteria are included in the study management protocol.

Summary
Selected discussions of research design features were presented. These are valuable in assisting the investigator to *think about* research, both in general and in specific terms.

Chapter 4

Research Planning

Introduction

The research plan describes the capture and utilization of information and gives a detailed structural and procedural description of the observations to be obtained. The plan is also an expression of the value of the investigation. Elements involved in the planning process are

1. identification of the existing facts and theories
2. translation of the concepts involved to related measurement sets
3. formation of hypotheses through rearrangement of the measurement sets
4. evaluation of the hypotheses in terms of relevance, innovation, and feasibility.

Identification

The identification element includes the review, evaluation, and organization of the various sources of information. This "literature review" is intended to yield an up-to-date body of knowledge of the subject.

Figure 4.1 illustrates the complexity of this literature review process. Journals, books, and reports are the basic sources reviewed first to select the most useful information. Computerized retrieval systems employing *keywords* to use in matching requests with stored material is an example of this activity. These manuscripts, abstracts, and other sources can be considered a reference file.

The cognitive processes involved in developing criteria for analysis of the documents in making decisions about retaining or discarding information are not identified and applied consistently. Attempts to formalize these involve either measurement or attribute detection rules about the choice of documents or the creation of a panel of judges to review the material.

Fig. 4.1.
The Literature Review Process.

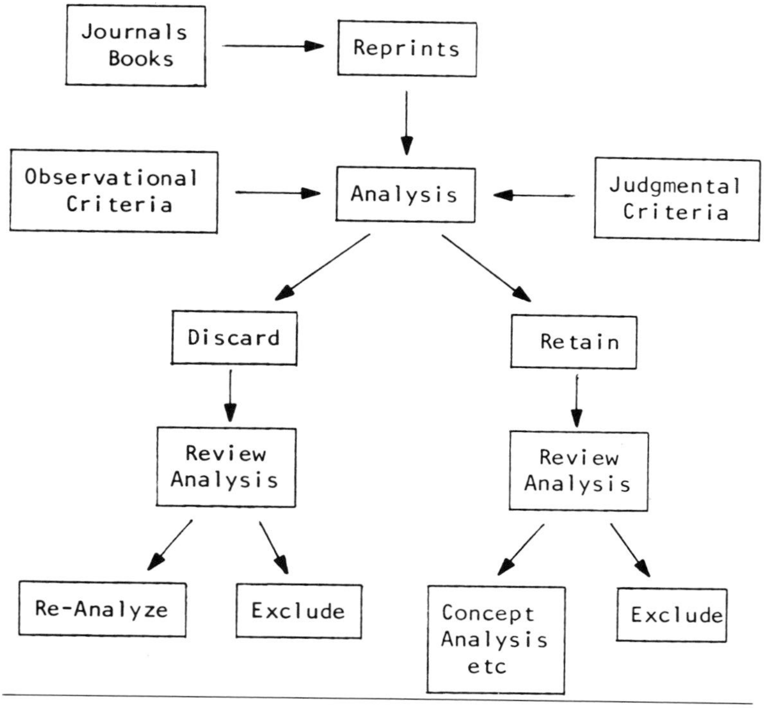

The first choice rests on the assumption that the cognitive process is used primarily to identify appropriate variates and to form criteria for selection. If this is accomplished, the measurements, analyses, and decision functions can be performed in a consistent and repetitive fashion. If a set of observations can be agreed upon, then the analysis may involve a traditional statistical format culminating in straightforward decision-making. The *observation* approach allows for reconsideration of the methods if excessive amounts of material are retained or discarded.

The use of panels of judges is best described by the Delphi Technique. In this approach, the panel members review the material independently. After each cycle of evaluation and decision, the members are made aware of the majority's decision and determine whether they agree or disagree with that decision. The pressure in the Delphi method is toward unanimous agreement. While minority views could persist, there is little incentive to do so since the individual members and the size of the minority are not revealed.

The functional process is

1. selection of material
2. separation of the set into retained and discarded material
3. identification of majority and minority decisions
4. review of discrepant material
5. separation of this material into the retained and discarded sets
6. identification of majority and minority decisions
7. . . .
8. . . .
9. . . .
10. final selection after stabilization of the panel's decision-making.

While the coordinators of a judgmental technique may speculate about the cognitive methods employed, it is clear that the members of the panel can invoke a variety of criteria in their decision-making which can vary with the membership of the group. Detection of those criteria can be frustrated by their variability. The advocates of these subjective group methods assume that experts will behave in a uniform and consistent fashion, thus allowing group membership and cycling variations to be discounted.

To illustrate the functions in the literature review-identification process, articles from a Sickle Cell Disease Symposium were used. The symposium was reported in the Archives of Internal Medicine (Lessin and Jensen 1974).

Review articles are of real value in the identification process. These articles frequently present the reader with a *list of keywords,* a *list of relationships* of interest, and an *outline of issues* considered by the expert to be relevant. As an example of this, some of the topics in the symposium were

1. genetic issues
2. rheological considerations
3. oxygen transport
4. hemolytic processes
5. coagulation issues
6. cardiovascular considerations
7. pulmonary complications
8. renal changes.

Key concepts from selected articles have been abstracted and are given in Table 4.1. These concepts will represent the reference file of documents.

As an example of the process shown in Figure 4.1, suppose that the criterion was the presence or absence of statistically significant data supporting the concept. That is, only those concepts *supported by data* and *by*

Table 4.1
Document File—Concepts

Area/Discipline	Concept
Genetics	A hemoglobin pattern showing a majority of the protein migrating as HbS cannot be accepted as proof that the person has sickle cell anemia.
	Other genotypes (S-β Thal., S-Dβ, and S-HPFH) also have a majority of protein migrating as HbS.
	Not all clinical expression of disease can be explained by the concomitant presence of known modifier genes.
	An understanding of the mechanisms of genetic modification may offer clues for effective therapy.
Rheology	Capillary blockage is associated with increased frequency of irreversibly sickled cells.
	Intravascular blood viscosity is a function of plasma viscosity, cellular components, red cell deformability, and vascular components.
	Plasma viscosity is a function of globulin concentration.
	Of the cellular components (red cells, platelets, leukocytes), the concentration of red blood cells is most important.
	The sickling distortion is the critical factor in red cell structure.
Oxygen Transport	Anemia could be considered in terms of blood oxygen delivery and not necessarily by hemoglobin content.
	By lowering the oxygen-hemoglobin affinity of the blood, compensation for reduced oxygen capacity or blood oxygen flow can occur. The clinical result is an asymptomatic cyanosis.
	An inverse relationship exists between size of sickled cells and the mean corpuscular hemoglobin concentration.
	Mean corpuscular hemoglobin also is related to the concentration of oxygen in the blood.
Coagulation	Vascular occlusion is initiated by the sickled erythrocytes by increasing blood viscosity and by promoting sludging in the capillaries and small venous channels.
	Chemical kinetics of thrombosis may be stimulated by the impeded blood flow.

significant results would be retained. This is an example of a simple *observational* approach where the observations are

1. concept supported by data and
2. data statistically significant.

The analysis could be designed to combine these results in a fashion

Table 4.2
Analysis of Concept Observations

Data Sets	Significance 2^2	+	Data 2^1	Result*
Neither	0		0	0
Data Only	0		1	2
Significance Only	—		—	—
Data and Significance	1		1	6

*Result $= x \cdot 2^1 + y \cdot 2^2$

where

$x = \{^0_1$, depicting presence or absence of data and
$y = \{^0_1$, depicting presence or absence of significance.

shown in Table 4.2. The analysis can be performed using binary arithmetic. The data are coded as 0 for absent or 1 for present. The concept requirements are ordered as follows:

1. data
2. significance.

The observational possibilities would yield scores of 0, 2, and 6.

The decision criterion could be to retain those concepts with a score of 6 and to discard those with scores of 0 or 2.

The review process at the bottom of Figure 4.1 could search for other reasons for retaining or discarding concepts. That is, a statistically based rationale may miss newer concepts not yet exposed to a sufficient number of tests for statistical assessment. For example, the four genetic concepts (Table 4.1) represent those which would be rejected using the observation-based analytical and decision criteria. These concepts would be retained by the review function. The rationale for retention might be that methods which describe hemoglobin patterns more definitively are a recent phenomenon. With these in use, there is need for additional studies and collection of test results. The larger number would then allow statistical evaluation.

The rheological concepts would be rejected by an observational analysis. They, too, might be retained by the review function as concepts too important to be discarded.

The oxygen transport and coagulation concepts would be retained by the analytical and decision criteria. On cognitive review, oxygen transport issues might be rejected because they contribute little to future study and are not fruitful. Similarly, the coagulation issues appear to be *a result* of the sickling process and therefore do not stimulate new studies.

This example of observational analysis and decision-making deals realist-ically with the complexities of sickle cell disease. In spite of the simple model used, it is clear that the method has merit. For example, the subjec-tive review emphasized two additional attributes. These were

1. data were insufficient to decide
2. findings did or did not lead to new work.

With new areas of study, the issue of insufficient information is certainly important. As new technology surfaces, restudy of any area could result in the transient conclusion of insufficient data. Observational criteria thus should include opportunities for new input.

Other attributes offering potential for new information could also be trans-lated into specific observations identifying new relationships. Observations might be in the form of a question, such as, oxygen transport is related to coagulation: Yes or No? With a data record composed of such ques-tions, an analytical model similar to that shown in Table 4.2 could be con-structed. The ordering of questions might be in terms of preconceived importance or investigated analytically. The scores resulting from either approach would be organized into acceptance and rejection sets.

The expert panel approach to sickle cell disease has also been per-formed and is represented by a newly organized multi-institutional study. The Delphi technique was not employed. Instead, in a series of meetings, the investigators jointly reviewed and decided on the areas of study. With this format, the pressures of group dynamics could operate. The criteria used by this panel might have been to include all areas in the study which may be of interest. That is, eliminate *only* those areas of study which have been shown to be statistically and clinically insignificant.

In addition to reaching decisions, the panel method offers opportunity for involvement, for education, and for responsibility. These issues are impor-tant in motivating individuals to take on a study and to perform it with a high level of quality.

The two approaches can operate concurrently. The initial review shown in Figure 4.1 could have the measurement–analysis orientation. The second review could employ a panel technique. Criteria emerging from the panel could indicate measures of associated attributes and the review would shift from subjective to quantitative. This interactive process is at the center of functions such as data safety monitoring.

Translation to Measurements
A primary effort in science is to develop methods for more specific and accurate descriptions of the phenomenon under study. It is difficult to asso-ciate a theoretical construct to measurements. Failure to accomplish this leads to either the rejection of the concept or the rejection of the measure-

ment, depending on which is more firmly entrenched within the structure of the science.

For example, two descriptions of associations between phenotype and genotype are given. The first is shown in Table 4.3. The characteristics included are a partial list (see Konotey-Ahulu 1974). The phenotype may be composed of one or more specific measurements. The genotype is shown in terms of predominant hemoglobin abnormality. The frequency of the phenotype in that genotype group is given as a percentage. The percentages do not reflect mutually exclusive phenotypic characteristics. That is, an individual may present with one or more of the observable defects.

As seen in Table 4.3, 28% of patients with genotype SS had the hand-foot syndrome, thirteen percent had clubbing of fingers and toes, and three percent had aseptic necrosis of the femoral head. These manifestations of bone complications predominated in the SS genotype. Six percent of the SC genotype patients had aseptic necrosis.

Data given in Table 4.3 may be used to establish the initial concept of disorder. Such beginnings also typically use simple statistical models such as counting techniques. From these attempts, structures such as those shown in Figures 4.2 and 4.3 may be developed. Both figures identify as relevant the association between the concept (plasma viscosity), the measurements (fibrinogen, globulin), and the interpretation (cell-protein interaction). Quantitative data to express the information-relating concepts and measurements is shown in Figure 4.3. Concepts such as flow velocity,

Table 4.3
Selected Relationships Between Phenotype and Genotype in Sickle Cell Studies

	Genotype		
	SS	SC	S Thal
Phenotype	(Percent of Cases)		
Hand-Foot Syndrome	28	4	—
Bilirubin > 10 mg%	56	22	44
Aseptic Necrosis of Femoral Head	3	6	—
Chronic Ulcers above Medial Malleolus	11	2	—
Gnathopathy	32	12	—
Epistaxis	10	5	8
Priapism	3	1	—
Clubbing of Fingers or Toes	13	6	—

Fig. 4.2.
Relationship Between Concepts and Measurements.

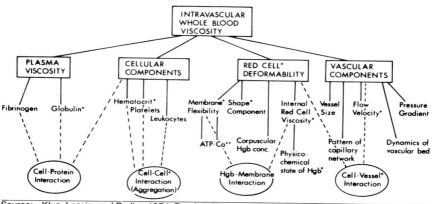

Source: Klug, Lessin, and Radice 1974. Reprinted by permission.

pressure gradient, and shear rate are expressed by values in different blood vessel systems. The concept and the measurement in Figure 4.3 assume the same label, though what is described is the concept rather than the device translating this to numbers. That is, as the measurement instrument improves technically, the label and the relationship between measurement and concept could remain unchanged.

An example of the attempt to improve the measurement process is illus-

Fig. 4.3.
Numeric Descriptions in Concept–Measurement Relationships.

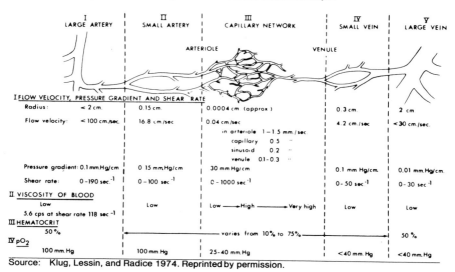

	I LARGE ARTERY	II SMALL ARTERY	III CAPILLARY NETWORK	IV SMALL VEIN	V LARGE VEIN
I FLOW VELOCITY, PRESSURE GRADIENT AND SHEAR RATE					
Radius:	< 2 cm.	0.15 cm	0.0004 cm (approx.)	0.3 cm.	2 cm.
Flow velocity:	< 100 cm./sec.	16.8 cm./sec	0.04 cm/sec in arteriole 1–1.5 mm./sec. capillary 0.5 " sinusoid 0.2 " venule 0.1–0.3 "	4.2 cm./sec	< 30 cm./sec.
Pressure gradient:	0.1 mm.Hg/cm	0.15 mm.Hg/cm	30 mm.Hg/cm	0.1 mm.Hg/cm.	0.01 mm.Hg/cm.
Shear rate:	0–190 sec.$^{-1}$	0–100 sec^{-1}	0–1000 sec^{-1}	0–50 sec^{-1}	0–30 sec^{-1}
II VISCOSITY OF BLOOD	Low 5.6 cps at shear rate 118 sec^{-1}	Low	Low ⟶ High ⟶ Very high	Low	Low
III HEMATOCRIT	50 %		varies from 10% to 75%		50 %
IV pO$_2$	100 mm.Hg	100 mm.Hg	25–40 mm.Hg	< 40 mm.Hg	< 40 mm.Hg

Source: Klug, Lessin, and Radice 1974. Reprinted by permission.

Table 4.4
More Specific Measurements of Hemoglobins (Genotypes) and Associations with Phenotypes

| | Genotypes | | | |
| | Hb A | Hb S | Hb A$_2$ | Hb F |
Phenotype	(%)	(%)	(%)	(%)
Normal	95–97	0	2–3	<2
Sickle Cell Trait	50–65	30–45	2–3	<2
Sickle Cell Anemia	0	75–95	2–4	<20
Sickle Cell Hb C	0	50–55	45–50*	<4
Sickle Cell Hb D β	0	95†	2–4	<5
S-HPFH	0	70–80	2–3	20–30

*Hb A$_2$ includes Hb C
†Hb S includes Hb D

trated in Table 4.4, which shows the relationship between phenotypes and genotypes using concentrations of the various hemoglobin moieties observed. As seen, the normal phenotype has potentially three forms of hemoglobin: Hb A ($\alpha_2\beta_2$); Hb A$_2$ ($\alpha_2\delta_2$); and Hb F ($\alpha_2\gamma_2$). The Hb A represents the pattern seen in normal persons and is made up of two genetic loci on the alpha and beta polypeptide chains. The altered molecule, Hb A$_2$, consists of two loci on the alpha chain and two on the delta chain. Fetal hemoglobin (Hb F) has two loci on the alpha chain and two on the gamma chain.

In contrast to the normal person with 95% to 97% of hemoglobin consisting of Hb A, those with either trait or disease have reduced amounts of Hb A and increases in other hemoglobin types. As seen, the individual with sickle cell trait has 30% to 45% of the total hemoglobin in the form of Hb S. Individuals with sickle cell anemia may vary in hemoglobin formation with a range of 75% to 95% consisting of Hb S. Those with persistent fetal hemoglobin have Hb S in concentrations of 70% to 80%, with 20% to 30% Hb F and 2% to 3% Hb A$_2$.

Depending on the measurement methods used, hemoglobin types may not be observed. This is seen in the sickle cell Hb C phenotype, where Hb A$_2$ and Hb C are included in the same location in a starch gel electrophoretic pattern. The cellulose acetate electrophoresis can be used to sort those genotypes involving Hb A, Hb S, and Hb C. In an analogous fashion, Hb D β may be differentiated from Hb S to reveal the distinction between sickle cell anemia and sickle cell Hb D β.

New Hypotheses

New hypotheses may be established by rearrangement and reorientation of measurement sets. Measurements are the key to relevance in describing the theoretical structure. When measurements satisfy the criteria of accuracy, reproducibility, and especially validity, the concepts comprising these measurements can be assessed for value. Those measurement-concept complexes of sufficient worth can be integrated into the structure describing the "state of the art."

The relationships between concepts and measurements shown in Figure 4.2 are integrated into a more global picture in Figure 4.4. Figure 4.4 delineates the shape factors, viscosity issues, coagulation, and hematopoietic processes which form the vaso-occlusive episode. This event is frequently associated with sickle cell crisis.

Specific hypotheses may be formed from such a picture. Examples of a few are given in Table 4.5, with the measurements included. In inspecting these hypotheses, the reader should identify the translations from concept(s) to related measurements (often called the dependent variates), to criterion measurements or observations (the independent

Fig. 4.4.
A Broader Theoretical Structure.

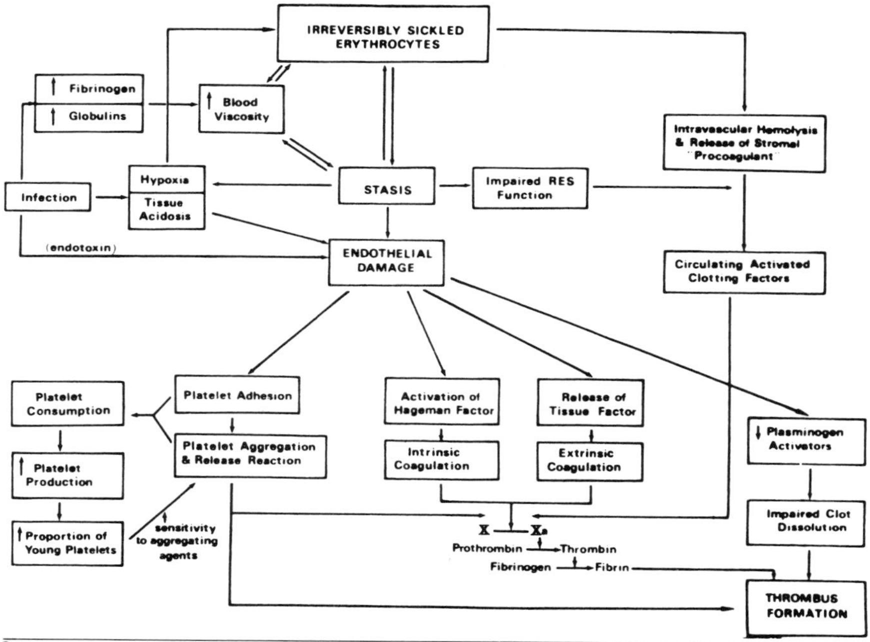

Source: Rickles and O'Leary 1974. Reprinted by permission.

Table 4.5
Hypotheses from the Structure Given in Figure 4.4

		Measurements	
Hypothesis	**Selection**	**Independent**	**Dependent**
Blood viscosity is a function of change in globulin.	All genotypes	Globulin	Flow velocity
The presence of irreversibly sickled cells "caused" thrombus formation.	Genotypes with Hb S and no Hb A	Percent of cells—ISC	Presence of clot; or concentration of thrombin, fibrin, platelets, etc.
Endothelial damage is a function of infection, hypoxia, tissue acidosis, and stasis.	Patients with ISC	Presence of infection, tissue hypoxia, tissue acidosis, and stasis	Pain, swelling, etc.

variates), and to selection variates which define the environment and/or population in the study. These variates and relationships are designed to assess the veracity of the hypothesis. This relationship among the measurements and observations is shown in Figure 4.5.

The *selection* variates (Figure 4.5) represent those observations and measurements which are believed to have a significant influence on the concepts, so that the results should be considered within each group selected. In terms of study design, the investigation would be replicated within each defined group. This approach allows assessment of the influence of the selection variates.

Fig. 4.5.
Measurement Types and Functions in Study Design.

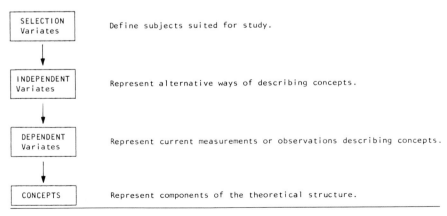

SELECTION Variates — Define subjects suited for study.

INDEPENDENT Variates — Represent alternative ways of describing concepts.

DEPENDENT Variates — Represent current measurements or observations describing concepts.

CONCEPTS — Represent components of the theoretical structure.

The *independent* and *dependent* variates represent the essence of the hypothesis, in that the question *always* posed is the existence of a relationship between the independent and dependent sets. The dependent variates are assumed to represent the concepts in an explicit, direct fashion. The independent ones could be potential substitutes for the dependent variates.

Evaluation

Hypotheses to study could be selected from the potentially long list by using the criteria of relevance, innovation, and feasibility. Feasibility is the easiest to assess. The questions to be answered are simply

1. *Can the procedures be accomplished for an individual subject in a timely and cost-effective fashion? And*

2. *Can these procedures be accomplished, again in a timely and cost-effective fashion, when replicated for each individual to be studied?*

A frequent concern in feasibility assessment is the availability of study subjects. "Guesstimates" often determine beginning sample sizes. However, records documenting the entry of desired individuals usually exist and can be analyzed. This effort in planning offers psychological and physical advantages. The *security* of factual material should not be discounted. Knowledge of the accrual rate and size factors associated with the study can be used to document the needs for improvement in facilities and to support staffing changes and task redefinitions. Step by step description and analysis are the means by which the feasibility questions posed above may be answered. The diagrams in Chapter 3 can assist the investigators in achieving appropriate analytical descriptions of their intended studies.

The *newness* of the study can be judged in a relatively straightforward fashion. The questions to be answered are

1. *Are the groups or environments studied new?*

2. *Are the methods used new?*

3. *Are the measurements new?*

4. *Are the concepts new?*

Answers to these questions also provide insight into the relevance of the study. Clearly, the recency and originality of the concepts studied can be a measure of the importance of the work. However, simple novelty is not sufficient.

If the concepts are not new, are the measurements new? The search continues for specific, accurate, reproducible, real world indicators of theoretical issues. If new measurements are found, the importance of the study is enhanced.

Fig. 4.6.
Collapse of a Theoretical Structure to a Relevant Hypothesis.

Hemoglobin
   Types

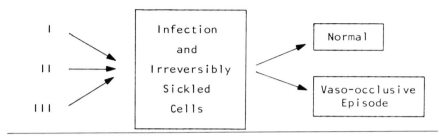

Methodological improvements in obtaining measurements are of technological interest but the "science" is normally not affected by these improvements. Extensions of previous concepts, measurements, and methods to
new populations is of secondary importance. These studies may produce
unexpected and exciting results and modify the theoretical constructs in
important ways. However, the typical pattern of effort does not lead to new
ideas. Instead, the catalog of established processes expands to include
the new group.

Indicators of *relevance* must, therefore, include originality and significance. When possible, the statements which offer the greatest potential for
collapsing an established elaborate structure into a simple one are the *most
important.* For example, the statement that the *vaso-occlusive episode*
was a *specified function* of *only infection and irreversibly sickled cells* in
patients with *particular patterns* of *hemoglobin types* would reduce the
description in Figure 4.4 to that shown in Figure 4.6. If the simpler statement was both feasible (in terms of performance and accomplishment)
and employed new methods and measurements, its relevance would be
enhanced.

The primary issue is that the potentially most relevant study will be that
one (or small set) which *simplifies* the existing theoretical structure by:

1. replacing it
2. eliminating components of it, or
3. replacing complex components with simpler ones.

Summary
Research planning consists of four areas of cognition and behavior. These
are

1.   Identification of Existing Facts and Theories.

Procedures associated with the use of *keywords* to identify *complex disciplines* were discussed.

Two approaches were considered. The first was the *observational.* Measurements and / or attributes of the documents reviewed would be identified. A data record consisting of these characteristics would be prepared and a formal analysis performed.

The second approach employs expert judges to review and decide whether each document is to be retained. Identifying the criteria being employed by the judges may be part of the procedure.

2.   Translation of Concepts to Related Measurements.

Measurements must satisfy two criteria in order to be valuable as a descriptor. These are *accuracy* and *reproducibility.* In addition, the relationship between the concept and the measurement must be monotonic. This *validity* allows the measurement to *replace* the concept.

3.   New Hypotheses Through Rearrangement of Measurement Sets.

The assumption of a one-to-one relationship between measurements and concepts provides a means for testing new conceptual interactions with related measurements. This is a *trial and error* process.

4.   Evaluation of the Formal Hypotheses.

The criteria for deciding the potential value of these new hypotheses are (1) feasibility of accomplishment; (2) existence of "newness" in concepts, measurements, methods, or populations studied; (3) relevance of hypotheses in simplifying complex structures.

These ideas were illustrated using studies from sickle cell disease and related hemoglobinopathies.

Chapter 5

Information Processing

Introduction

Information processing is a composite technology whose methods origi-
nated in computer science, statistical analysis, and research methodology.
The need for this technology has increased with the growth of multi-
disciplinary and multi-institutional research endeavors. The functions
included are

1. Data Processing
   a. data record construction
   b. data file construction
   c. data validation procedures
2. Data Management
   a. data form construction
   b. data monitoring procedures
   c. data displays
   d. data analyses
3. Protocol Management
   a. protocol development
   b. staff training and orientation
   c. simulation studies
4. Program Management
   a. concepts and related measurements
   b. protocol performance procedures
   c. scientific and educational material.

Data Processing

Data processing is the most mechanical and elementary function. The basic
intention is to transform the observations and measurements into readable
and manageable computer records.

Data processing alone can do much to transform data into new issues. For example, in one research center, admission data have been recorded on data forms and then keypunched. A program was prepared which *collated* separate admissions for an individual patient, *sorted* these admissions by date, and *listed* the dates with the admission diagnoses. These relatively simple listings were used to check accuracy and to assess procedural problems. The listings drew attention to the need to review diagnostic criteria. With suitable review and reporting procedures, patients who became eligible for special studies, as their characteristics and measurements changed, could be identified and reported to the participating investigators.

Data Management
Data management procedures are developed using two sources: specific scientific protocols, and general program requirements. General program requirements are a more basic, long-term approach to the information needs of a research program. The data captured would include such administrative issues as numbers of patients receiving various forms of health care. Also included would be demographic and epidemiologic issues such as the relationships between age, sex, psycho-social factors, survival and remission duration. Each of these could be related to the occurrence of "significant" medical events. These data would be obtained at entry and selected items would be repeated through time.

The data forms should, ideally, be incorporated into the health delivery process. Much of the data already exists in available hospital forms. These forms may be photocopied and relevant items abstracted by the data processing staff. This operation reduces to an absolute minimum the errors of repeated and redundant recording.

Since data monitoring includes the assessment of data records in terms of legibility, accuracy, and timeliness, the medical staff could review, correct, and clarify the hospital forms. Data not part of present hospital or outpatient processes, which represent desired segments of the long-term record, could be obtained by completion of specially prepared data forms. These forms would be constructed in conjunction with the involved investigators. The information processing staff would be responsible for providing procedural descriptions for data capture and reporting; for data review, both human and computer; for displays including the data; and for analyses describing the relationships anticipated among these and other data. Wherever possible, these special data records should be incorporated into the hospital record system to reduce the aura of special investigation and to establish one of mandatory routine, recording, and reporting.

Protocol Management
The scientific thrust of a multidisciplinary research program implies a continuing process of protocol development, conduct, and closure. These proto-

cols may deal with questions confined to a single laboratory as well as ones requiring a multidisciplinary approach. Accordingly, different mechanisms must be available to provide support both to the single investigator and to interdisciplinary teams. Protocol development for basic investigations may be one of acting as a "sounding board," assisting the investigator to formalize his ideas, arrange his priorities, and construct data record keeping which allows periodic analyses. This interactive process provides essential information for the types and schedules of anticipated studies.

Assistance in multi-disciplinary protocol development usually requires a more formal document to insure that the principals agree to perform the "same study." This more detailed plan contains criteria for:

1. eligibility of patients
2. study measurements and observations
3. study therapies
4. surveillance measurements
   a. toxicities
   b. disease complications
   c. disease resolution
5. study management assessment
6. study results reporting.

The protocol serves as the basis for both preparation of data management procedures and for staff orientation.

The information processing staff, to fulfill their role in protocol management, must perform two additional tasks. The protocol must be initially reviewed and tested for feasibility. This testing process may take many forms, from computer simulation to performance of pilot studies.

With the protocol in final form, a critical step prior to initiation is staff orientation. The number of persons involved in the conduct of a clinical or clinical-laboratory study is frequently underestimated until samples fail to appear or appear unexpectedly. Identifiying participants and preparing appropriate descriptive material is an important service provided by the information processing staff.

Program Management
Many research centers distinguish their programs by assigning priorities to concepts to be studied. Scientific concepts change as do their relationship to one another, and to the measurements used to translate the concepts to real events. An important service provided by the information processing unit is the description of current studies and findings pertinent to the conceptual structure under study. A simple mechanism to do this would include:

1. measurements involved (biochemical description of hemoglobinopa-

thies, pulmonary functions, liver functions, rheological characteristics), and

2. time data (date started, estimated completion date, dates of reports, manuscripts, and publications).

The communications explaining the program should be prepared by the information processing staff. These invariably include scientific and educational material. This effort aids in determining the program's direction and outcome. Included in this evaluation are the assessments of individual protocols and of the format of the core data capture process. Much of this has taken place, in the past, around the preparation of progress reports for funding agencies. The staff can employ techniques to make this evaluation possible on a current basis.

Scientific Concepts and Information Processing

Information utilization involves the identification of concepts. When this has been done, appropriate measurements related to these concepts may be selected and the testing process initiated (see Chapter 4). For example, in sickle cell studies, the most important concept is the existence of a distribution of hemoglobin moieties. A large number of mutants have been detected which include all of the various polypeptide chains. In contrast with older classifications using the predominant hemoglobin to characterize the individual, it is now preferable to include all of the forms identified and to record the percent of the individual's total hemoglobin represented by each structural entity. For example, normal individuals might be characterized as 95 to 97% Hb A, 0% Hb S, 2 to 3% Hb A_2, and less than 2% Hb F. In contrast, the patient with sickle cell anemia might be evaluated relative to these concentrations. That is, the non-crisis period may be associated with the lower amounts of Hb S (i.e., the 75% level) and the crisis period with the higher amounts (95% level). The question studied could be, "Does this concentration vary in prognostic relationship to crisis?"

Formulation and arrangement of the selected concepts and measurements may suggest studies designed to supply answers in a relatively short period of time. Other hypotheses may require longer periods to accumulate sufficient numbers of patients and to allow each patient to evolve (or resolve) the disease process.

Short-Term Studies

Short-term scientific endeavors derive from succinct arrangements of the concepts and may be characterized in terms of the measurements included, the timing of data capture, and the analytical results anticipated. The measurement sets are classified as:

1. selection
2. independent
3. dependent.

The *selection* variates represent those observations and measurements which are believed to have a significant influence on the concepts, so that the results could be different within each group of individuals selected. These variates include those indicating eligibility for a particular study *and* significant front-end variability.

The *independent* and *dependent* variates represent the essence of the hypothesis studied, in that the question *always* posed is the existence of a relationship between the measurements termed independent and those called dependent. The dependent ones are *assumed* to represent the concepts in an explicit, direct fashion. The independent ones are potential substitutes for the dependent ones.

Examples of this relationship are shown in Figures 5.1 and 5.2. In Figure 5.1, age is the independent variate and first episode of splenomegaly is the dependent variate. In Figure 5.2, age is the independent variate, severe infection is the dependent variate, and groups defined in terms of age at first evidence of splenomegaly are the selection variates.

A number of such studies may be formulated. For example, consider a study which seeks to describe the relationship between percentage of Hb S and its change in concentration with crisis. The selection variates might be one or more of the following:

1. crisis
2. age
3. sex
4. concentration of Hb F.

The independent variate might be maximum change in Hb S during period prior to crisis. The dependent variate might be the time to episode.

Only patients with an episode of crisis would be included. Subgroupings might be considered employing age, sex, or Hb F. The measurements of hemoglobin distribution, and of maximal change in concentration of Hb S, would be available. The graphs would be similar to those shown in Figure 5.3. The study groups would be: (1) no change in Hb S concentration; (2) decrease in concentration; and (3) increase in concentration. *If* individuals experience crisis with either *no change* or *decreased concentration of Hb S,* the time span to crisis is expected to be longer than for those who show an increase in concentration of Hb S.

Long-Term Studies
These represent a research program's core questions relating front-end factors such as age, sex, and initial hemoglobin distribution to significant clinical events. The data would be gathered to serve a variety of immediate and long-term requirements.

The data and the planned analyses would be restricted to those needed for the basic set of relevant long-term questions.

Fig. 5.1.
Survival Curve Indicating First Appearance of Splenomegaly (n = 135).

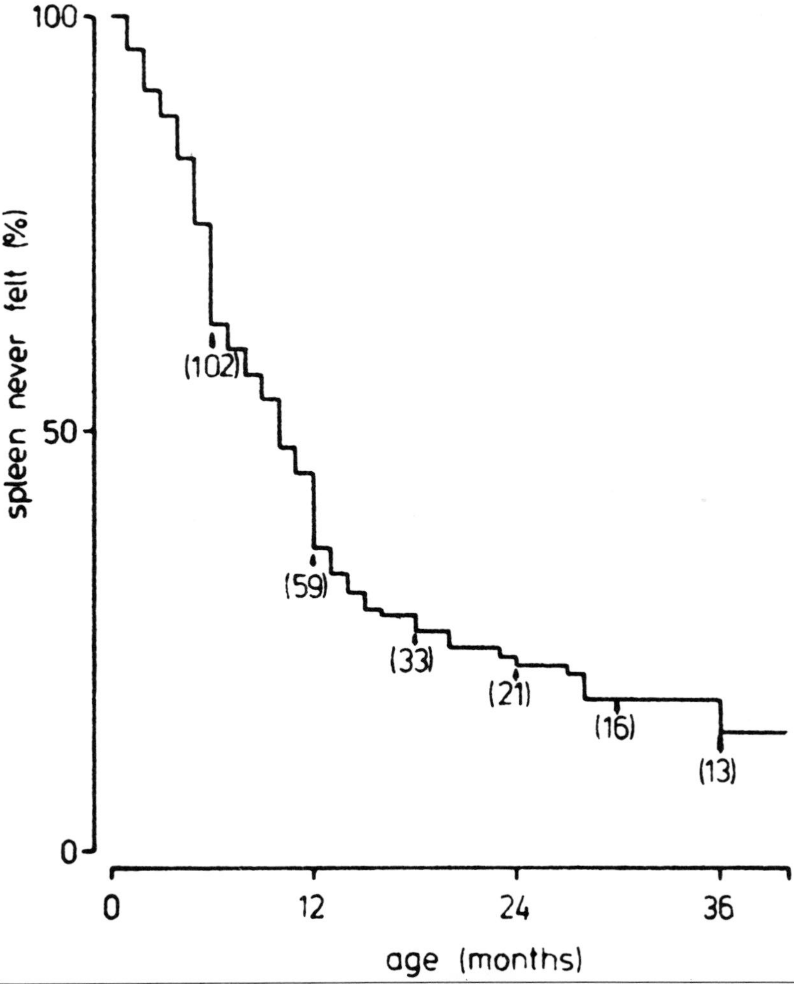

Source: Rogers, Vaidya, and Serjeant 1978. Reprinted by permission.

For example, the data record in a long-term sickle cell disease study might include

1. age at entry
2. sex
3. psycho-social factors
4. first admission diagnosis and time of event
5. first serious diagnosis and time of event

6. number of separate admissions
7. minimum time interval between admissions
8. maximum time interval between admissions
9. total disease-free interval
10. first specific diagnosis (e.g., crisis) and time of event
11. maximum disease-free interval between episodes of specific
    diagnosis
12. survival status and duration.

Fig. 5.2.
**Survival Curves Representing Pattern of First Severe Infection According
to Spleen Groups.**

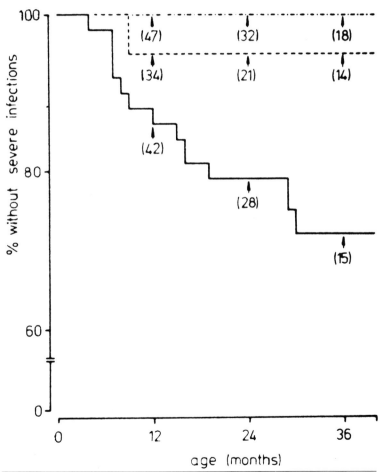

Source: Rogers, Vaidya, and Serjeant 1978. Reprinted by permission.

Fig. 5.3.
Hypothesized Outcomes.

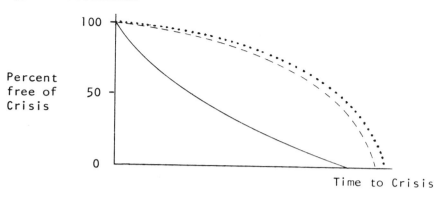

──── Increased Concentration

─ ─ Decreased Concentration

··· No Change

In addition to this set of multi-use data items, a set for eligibility definition might include first examination evaluation of:

1. Hb distribution
2. viscosity
3. oxygen transport
4. hemolysis
5. clotting
6. cardiovascular status
7. pulmonary status
8. renal status
9. hepatic status
10. infection experience.

The set might also include maximal change and timing associated with either regular physical examinations or with hospital admissions for disease.

As implied, these data would make it possible to

1. classify individuals using first observations during a "well" period
2. detect change in these parameters with illness, and
3. categorize the changes with respect to disease entities experienced.

With ensuing subgroups of patients, short-term studies could investigate relationships among newer measures as they became identified.

Procedural Details in Providing an Information Processing Service

A number of procedural elements which constitute the complete support process associated with effective information utilization are described in this section.

Data Record Construction

The initial vehicle for computerized data handling may be the punched card. This is prepared by identifying and copying the data from either existing hospital/outpatient records or from forms created by the Center staff.

Punched cards may be prepared as requested by investigators or as data summaries become available. This *ad hoc* approach can and does lead to the typical "peaks and valleys" of over- and under-utilization of both staff and equipment.

Establishment of a formal schedule of studies would minimize problems in entering work tasks into the analytical queue. In order to expedite this orderly flow, the information processing unit should receive the form shown in Table 5.1 as early in the project development and execution process as possible.

As seen, this simple notification mechanism, completed by the responsible investigator, documents the necessary interactions between the staff required to punch, verify, read, list, and organize the data for analysis; the staff required to review the scientific goals of the project and to translate those into appropriate analyses; and the participating researchers (or health care providers) who interpret the analyses and use the information derived.

Data File Construction

Data files may serve various purposes, such as:

1. basic storage (archival)
2. interim or holding file (temporary repository before permanent storage or translation to analyses)
3. analytical (temporary repository discarded after analysis completed).

A new data set must be classified in terms of its short-term and long-term file structure.

An important component of the data processing supervision is an inventory describing the existing data files and their interrelationships. This inventory should be available for continuing review by the investigators. The following information should be displayed:

Table 5.1
Data Preparation Alert Form

Project: _____

Investigator: _____

Data Ready to Punch: ___(anticipated date)_____

Analyses Defined: ___(consultation referral number)_____

Analysis Due Date: ___(anticipated date)_____

1. measurement set (Hb distribution, blood viscosity parameters, etc.)
2. patient subgroup (crisis only *and* age 1–3 years, etc.)
3. time frame (from specific date to specific date)
4. file type (*archival, entry* or holding prior to permanent storage, *retrieval* or holding prior to translation for analyses, *analytical* or temporary)
5. analyses employed (life table, histograms, etc.—consultation referral number may be used in lieu of analytical codes)
6. status (presently used—Y/N).

Data Validation

In usual "batch" efforts, the data are abstracted from primary records, copied onto "coding" forms, keypunched, and verified. That is, the keypunch operation is validated. The initial data abstraction and copy process may or may not be verified. In a dynamic program, involving continuing abstraction of primary records with data recording and reporting, the initial portion may not be validated since fatigue and related error issues are considered minimal.

The importance and expense of the study mandates the information processing unit to monitor quality control in documenting data abstraction and reporting accuracy. General sampling plans to be used might be

1. For small "batch" data sets (less than 50 records), total abstraction and recording could be performed by a second reviewer. The two data sets could be compared and a corrected set obtained.
2. For large "batch" data sets (over 50 records), a random sampling plan could be established. Criteria for data acceptance would include procedures for multi-stage sampling, in order to estimate the proportion of error. Depending upon the error observed and the scheduling constraints, the investigators will decide final acceptance or rejection of the data set. Rejection would require a complete second abstraction and comparison of the two sets to obtain a correct one.
3. For continuing data reporting, a random sampling of data records, blocked by time, would be a minimum quality control monitoring

technique. If observed error statistics changed in defined ways, larger independent samples would be taken.

These sampling plans require a second independent abstraction and reporting of the data. In addition, the data processing unit should produce data displays which could be used in lieu of the primary records. That is, if laboratory data were abstracted from the original report forms, a summary record representing the experience for that patient might be displayed as shown in Table 5.2.

The display integrates the new data record with the previously reported material and provides an "updated" description of the identified parameters. The form provides the staff with the opportunity to validate the entire record as well as the last entry. In addition, the form shows evidence that the data are used.

Data Form Construction
The process of recording data is intimately related to the original capture. In many ways, the data form guides the capture process. These pragmatic considerations are particularly relevant when scientific investigations are coupled with health care.

One approach in establishing the link is to create new primary data recording forms which can store the entire information base for the project. These forms could replace the usual hospital / outpatient forms and thus become the primary documents.

A second way is to create project-related primary data forms. These are completed either at the same time as the hospital forms or shortly thereafter. The source of information is the observer rather than the primary hospital records.

Table 5.2
Display of Reorganized Data

Patient Identification: _____

Date	BUN	Total Bilirubin	Cholesterol	Pro-Time	Control
760101	20	.6	200	95%	11 sec.
760601	19	.5	210	96%	10 sec.
761201	22	.3	205	98%	11 sec.
770210	20	.7	220	99%	11 sec.
.	.	.	.	.	.
.	.	.	.	.	.

A third way is to create project-related data abstraction forms. These use the primary hospital records as the source. Missing data are frequent and may limit number and scope of analyses.

A fourth approach is a combination of project-related primary data forms and data abstraction forms. This method offers the advantage of continuing interaction with the clinical team involved in recording primary data. The missing data problem may be reduced, due to this closer participation between investigators and health care providers.

An important consideration for the investigators and the information processing unit of a new project is the source of the data. Investigators tend to create a new document containing all of the required data, even when that form is a simple restructuring of other forms. Copying, sorting, collating, and listing are performed accurately by computers. Creating the new data forms may therefore be unnecessary.

When new data forms are needed, they should be integrated into the usual data capture process as closely as possible. Steps in preparing data forms include

1. identification of the observations and measurements required
2. arrangement into sets associated with the processes of data capture
3. development of criteria for evaluating the immediate acceptability of the characteristic
4. development of criteria for necessary, immediate classification of patients, based on the values of observations and measurements
5. simulation of the capture and evaluation processes
6. independent testing using staff in the data capture environment
7. identification of potential analyses including the measurements or observations
8. final assessment of "worth" in problem resolution.

The importance of the data form lies in the information potential. Discussions between investigators and statistical and data processing staff should lead to satisfaction of the following goals:

1. minimal creation of new data forms
2. maximal utilization of primary records for abstraction and preparation of computer records
3. maximal utilization of existing computer records to develop new analytical records and files, and
4. maximal prereview and recognition of information potential for analyses and interpretation.

Data Monitoring

The monitoring of the data reflecting the patient's progress is an obvious issue in data management. This is usually performed manually by the health care providers or investigators. The information processing unit should ascertain, for each new project, the potential usefulness in instituting computer-supported monitoring. These procedures will increase costs as well as information potential. If investigators are resistant to these supports, the costs cannot be justified, as the information will not be used.

Study progress should be monitored. Issues such as patient (sample) accrual, adverse events, beneficial events, schedule adherence, and information derived are important, of mutual concern, and should be regularly updated and available to the investigative group.

Details of data monitoring which involve accuracy of observations were discussed in the Data Validation section.

Data Displays
Two principal forms should be available on a regular basis. Patient displays are an example of new data form contruction, when the new represents restructuring of existing data. A display of patient data allows for continuing review of accuracy of the elements and provides by inference the set of questions involved in collection of new data. These two processes, review and addition, form a key element in the larger process of information use.

The other form of data display is the graphic analysis. Usual ones are histograms, cumulative frequency graphs (e.g., life table type), and bivariate scatter diagrams. These displays should be designed at the outset of the study, so that data preparation, analysis, and reporting may be scheduled into the data processing and management work queue.

Data Analyses
In the study preparation period, emphasis on data analysis often seems incomprehensible as well as irrelevant. However, the analytical models to be used determine the sample size requirements as well as the extent of the information to be observed. No additional insight is possible *after* data analysis. Review of the measurement set, with simulation and exploration of suitably formulated hypotheses, will give the investigator a range of anticipated data results. From that review, the joint task of the investigators and information processing staff is to identify those analyses which will assist in describing the realized data results. These models should be identified, programmed, and incorporated into the computer process for that study. Some statisticians believe that the models should be used from the outset of the study, even before the sample sizes or the events warrant *appropriate* use.

Protocol Development
The protocol defines the procedures involved in accomplishing the intended work. In scientific endeavors, these work tasks tend to be classified as:

1. Developmental
   a. A measurement procedure is specified and undergoes technical review and stabilization.
   b. A potential therapy is identified and biological response data are gathered using animals as the test subjects.

2. Evaluative
   a. The established measurement procedure is now employed in a variety of settings, in order to establish its usefulness relative to existing standards.
   b. The potentially useful therapy is explored in a variety of patient types, in order to establish conditions of its usefulness relative to existing forms of therapy for like illnesses.

3. Service
   a. This may consist of routine laboratory and / or clinical functions and data. When added to the scientific data, these provide more complete descriptions of the patient's status at entry and throughout the study. The protocol should contain descriptions of the collection and processing of these service-related elements. Alternatively, the scientific activity itself may be a service. This is a common experience in laboratories engaged in developing and testing new procedures. The health care provider may collaborate with the laboratory to expand the usual description of a patient's status.

Clearly, the study design requirements change with the task to be accomplished. However, the following would usually be obtained from the investigator:

1. Measurements to be Used
   a. concept area (e.g., Hb characteristics, viscosity parameters, etc.)
   b. status of measurements (e.g., developmental, evaluative, service)
   c. use in proposed study (e.g., selection, independent, dependent sets)

2. Relationships Anticipated
   a. differences
   b. correlations

3. Timing
   a. data capture
   b. data records available
   c. analytical reports due.

Using answers to the above as a beginning, the investigators and information processing staff could develop the dialogue necessary for a concise and complete description of the intended work. This document would be circulated to data processing, data management, and to those interested in the scientific review process. When compiled, the protocol would contain the design elements, sample size requirements, data procedures, and analytical implications.

Staff Training
The protocols in operation, the organizational structure, and the reports from the projects constitute the raw material for orienting new personnel. Furthermore, as each new protocol becomes available, the appropriate staff must be trained. There must be evidence of understanding and intention to comply with the protocol procedures.

Simulation
This trial process is an important component in the development of new protocols and in the orientation of staff. The results of the simulation can identify defects in structure and in operation. Staff involvement in the simulation process is a valuable form of training.

Summary
The procedures included in information processing have been described.

One of the principal advantages of the single-institution multi-disciplinary research structure is the geographical proximity of the individuals involved. Much of the information processing support in planning can be accomplished through discussion. The specifics of interest to the investigator can, in this way, be identified and resolved.

As the distance between the individuals increases, such as in multi-institutional cooperative research programs, the techniques themselves become more relevant. There is the continuing task of transforming a general method into specific procedures to be used in the study. This technique may be learned so it can be replicated by individuals with the relevant training. Information processing as a composite technology incorporates computer science, statistics, and research methodology. The specific methods which transform ideas into measurement sets and then to analyses may be identified and "borrowed" from the primary disciplines.

Chapter 6

Analysis of Functions

Introduction

The patient management protocol is the basic blueprint for the sequence of procedures, staffing needs, and informational elements. This guide, when coupled with the following graphic techniques, provides the investigator with a simple, straightforward approach to describing and evaluating the clinical research to be performed.

Functions and Behavior

The symbols used in the graphic description have been standardized, so that the same general functions apply to each of the symbols.

There are seven basic behaviors which coincide to complete an action. This *act,* or behavior module, is accomplished through the sequence shown in Figure 6.1. That is, given that the intellectual activities (cognitive function) and the resulting selection of criteria were accomplished, the behavior begins with a *contact* or a communication. Information in the form of measurements or observations is collected through this contact. These data are stored in a repository. Storage and retrieval are accomplished using the appropriate filing criteria and procedure. The data, once retrieved, become available for analysis, and application of the analytical model leads to a decision. Subsequent actions repeat this sequence of behaviors / functions.

The module of behavior is a convenient mnemonic for describing key parts of the research process. Since the sequence of functions shown in Figure 6.1 occurs in each specific act, the investigator can formulate the total research effort by linking these modules. Further, the investigator can supply complete descriptions by matching each part with the associated symbol. This permits agreement between the specific behavior, the general function, and the corresponding symbol.

Fig. 6.1.
The Behavioral Module.

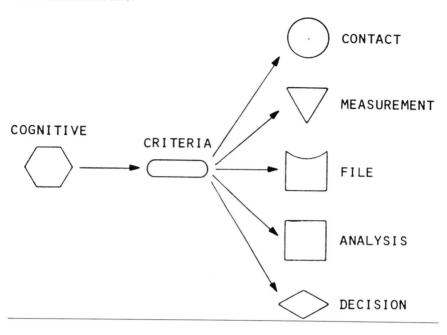

Functional Analysis and Physical Examination

The descriptive capability of this graphic approach is illustrated by the physical examination in Figure 6.2. The contact functions include interview, inspection, . . . percussion. For each contact, individual characteristics are observed and are recorded onto various forms (files). The purpose of the analyses is the assessment of normality. These individual findings are integrated to describe the person's health status.

In Figure 6.3 activity is differentiated according to "who" performs the function. The contact function is performed by the physician and by the technicians (laboratory, ECG, X-ray, clinical, etc.). Similarly, the measurement function is divided into those measurements obtained by the physician, and those measurements obtained by the technician. The measurements obtained by the physician are used to decide questions of normality for each characteristic considered. In contrast, the measurements obtained by the technician are permanent and may be used repeatedly by the same or different physicians when an analysis of the total findings is performed. The distinction in measurement activities can be clarified by the following example.

The physician, when asked to consider the size and shape of the head, may determine a number of measurements, all being estimated by observa-

Fig. 6.2.
Functional Description of the Physical Examination.

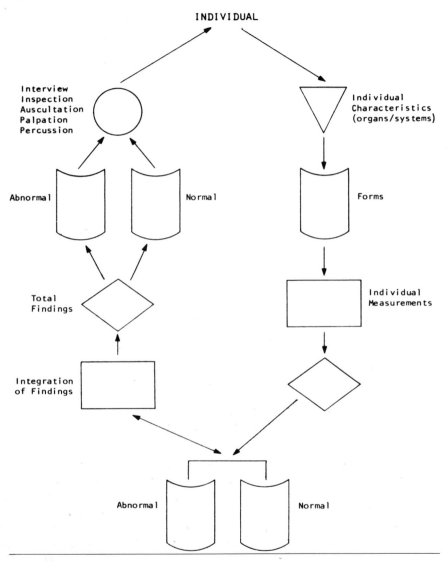

tion. That is, none of these characteristics are measured with appropriate instruments, nor are these measurements recorded as separate events. Such measurements may include, for example, the size of each part or the angular relationships between the parts. These measurements are *observed* by the physician, *immediately analyzed,* and a *decision* as to normal or abnormal shape and size is recorded.

Fig. 6.3.
Personnel Relationships.

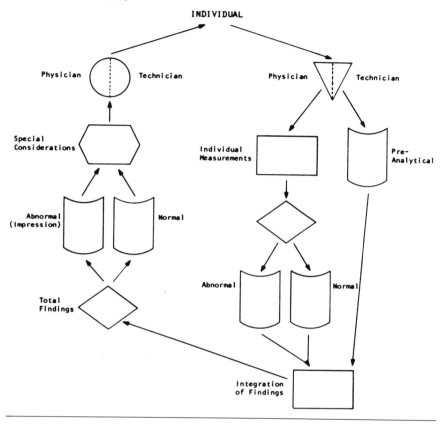

In contrast, the technician, when asked to measure the size and shape of the head, will use instruments such as tape measure, calipers, camera, X-ray. These instruments, when used according to *specific criteria,* will give measurements which are reproducible. If photographic or X-ray records are obtained, measurements from these permanent documents may be obtained any number of times. The instrument generating the measurement does not involve human perceptions directly, but rather some physical characteristic, and, accordingly, these measurements have been denoted as *objective.* The advantages of objective measurements are: (1) they are reproducible; (2) they have relatively less variation; (3) they are cheaper, in that the training of technicians is considerably shorter than that of physicians and technician's time is less expensive; (4) they are permanent compared to those obtained and used by the physician; and (5) they tend to be numerical and to incorporate a larger range of numbers than those observed by the physician and hence are capable of greater categorization.

Fig. 6.4.
Separation of Duties.

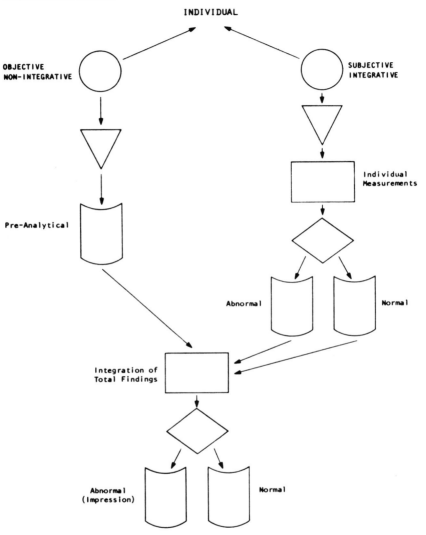

These two kinds of contact-measurements used in the physical examination representing two distinctively different processes are identified
in Figure 6.4. The first, performed by the technician, requires an objective
measurement made through a non-integrative process. The second is
performed by the physician who employs his faculties to obtain the measurements, to analyze the situation and to make decisions. This has been
denoted as the subjective-integrative process. A second important point

also demonstrated in Figure 6.4 is the analytical function the physician used in integrating all of the findings. This analysis represents the meaningful cognitive effort employed by the physician. In performing this function, he utilizes his training and experience in determining the ultimate proper category in which the examined individual belongs. This analytical function identifies, combines, weighs, and evaluates the total measurement set and establishes the appropriate summaries for the decision-making function. This analytical-decision process represents the major result of the physical examination from which appropriate actions will or will not be taken.

It is clear that greater emphasis should be placed on the physician's performance of the analytical-decision process. If the physical examination were based on the objective, non-integrative process performed by technicians, it would yield permanent, efficient measurements and would free the physician from the measurement function, enabling him to intensify his analytical role.

Functional Analysis in Clinical Studies

The module shown in Figure 6.1 and the overview sequences shown in Figures 6.2 through 6.4 demonstrate the potential for describing complex processes by grouping all like functions. All of the contact functions can be grouped and described by one symbol (the circle) as can the other functions. The questionnaire shown in Table 6.1 is an aid in this identification

---

Table 6.1
Specific Questions Leading to a Functional Analysis of the Problem

1. List every contact you can think of. Do not concern yourself with the appropriate order yet.

2. For each contact listed, what information is *sent* or *received?*
   Record answers in same order as 1.

3. Where is the information stored? For each contact, list the file for each piece of information.

4. What analyses are performed using each information set? Specifically indicate whether the information is *edited* for completeness, extreme values, and logical discrepancies; analyzed for *differences;* analyzed for *relationships;* analyzed for *evidence of reproducibility;* analyzed for *evidence of variability.*

5. What decisions are made as a result of the analyses? List for each.

6. Where are these decisions stored?

7. What functions indicated above give rise to the need for non-routine, higher level intervention, that is, identify the steps needing special human considerations?

8. For each function above, list the specific criteria which have been developed.

9. Arrange these functions into an order which reflects desired flow of work, for example:

   Contact → Information → File → Analysis → Decision →
   File → Cognitive Action → Criteria → Contact . . . etc.

---

and grouping process. Each module is described by listing all of the control functions, simply maintaining the same order as answers to questions 1 through 8. The individual modules are organized and ordered in response to question 9. An alternative to the sequential flow in question 9 would be to rank and group the contents of each functional symbol.

The descriptive summary is illustrated in Figure 6.5 for a study designed to *survey* patients and normal persons. The purpose is to identify new attributes differentiating the two groups. This study design is called retrospective. Note that the complete process may be described in terms of a small number of functions and that the specific content of the function changes appropriately. For example, the initial contact is designed to recruit subjects for the study. The result of this contact is the identifying information which is recorded on a data sheet and filed. In addition to the identifying data, the subject's willingness to participate is noted. The file is reviewed (analyzed) and all subjects willing to participate are sent a letter (contact) and a simple health history form (measurement) for preliminary clinic screening. The returned forms are filed, analyzed for history of myocardial infarction or other major illness. If the subject reports a positive history and meets the required selection criteria (analysis), he is eligible for clinic examination

Fig. 6.5.
Summary of Retrospective Study—"What."

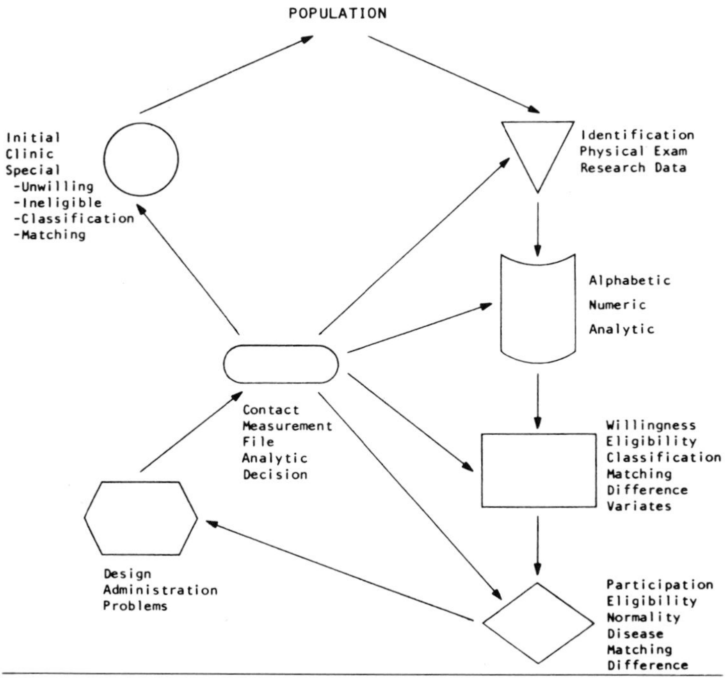

Fig. 6.6.
Retrospective Study—"How."

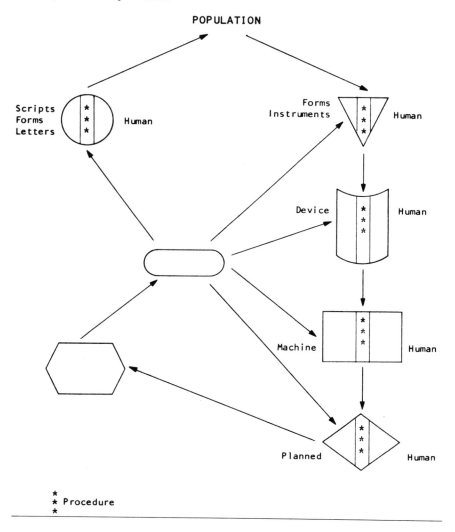

as a patient (decision). If the subject reports a negative history and meets
the required selection criteria (analysis), he is eligible for clinic as a possible normal subject (decision). The ineligible subjects (decision) receive
a letter (special considerations) thanking them for their willingness to participate, but indicating that they do not have the necessary qualifications for
the study.

As is seen from the symbolic representation, a number of specific questions related to proper procedures are immediately recognized. For exam-

Fig. 6.7.
Separation of Function: Human.

POPULATION

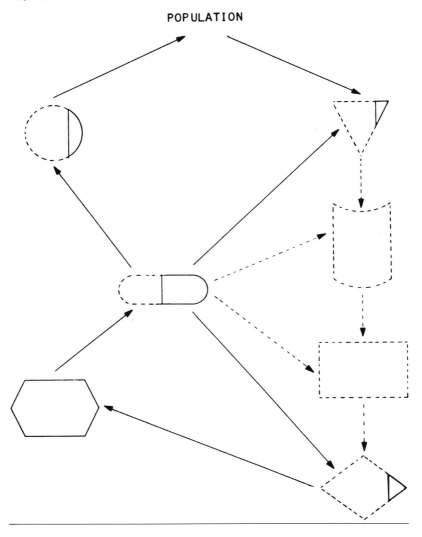

ple, the *cognitive function* identified at key spots in the program involves
questions of what to tell the unwilling person, the ineligible, or the un-
matched. Each procedure must clearly be specified, as to what to say on
initial contact, when to send the health screen, when and how many to
schedule for clinic, the type of clinical examination, the analyses to be
conducted, the laboratory methods, and so forth.

In Figure 6.6, the functions are analyzed in terms of *how* they are accomplished. As shown, each function may be subdivided into a human part, an instrument or form part, and a procedure part. Figure 6.5 shows *what is done* and Figure 6.6 shows *how it is done.*

At this point in the functional analysis, it should be emphasized that all functions may be performed *manually.* However, if one has the financial support, a number of improvements can readily be derived. We show this in Figure 6.7. For each function, certain aspects can best be performed by *humans.* We identify these in Figure 6.7 by a solid outline. In Figure 6.8, we have collected those parts of the functions which could be performed by a *machine.* The sum of the functions outlined in solid in Figures 6.7 and 6.8 are equivalent to those shown in Figure 6.6.

Functional Analysis and Scientific Method

As a final example of the ease in relating the symbolic description to behavioral processes, the flow events making up the scientific method are graphed. These are shown in Figure 6.9. Each discipline is a communication channel—a way of facilitating the flow of information and, thus, of perceiving the problem. We denote this function by the "circle" and label it as the *contact* function. The word, *contact,* was chosen to represent the notion that *perception* is possible only when the perceiver and the perceived establish a physical or psychological contact. This contact invokes the use of particular criteria which are created, modified, and abolished through the human *cognitive function* of interpretation and formalization.

Appropriate measurements must be obtained to study an environment. These measurements may depend on the use of human senses (subjective) or may stem from instruments based on physical characteristics (objective). The act of obtaining the measurement will depend on the criteria used. The resulting measurement may be stored according to various criteria in a file.

Three essential analyses are shown. These are

1. the identification of those measurements that are most *important* in describing or predicting the phenomenon studied

2. the comparison of pertinent measurements; that is, what information is obtained from *variate* A as compared with variate B?

3. the evaluation of pertinent measurements; that is, which of the pertinent measurements are better for *purpose* A as compared with purpose B?

On the basis of these analyses, decisions can be made. Examples of frequent decisions in either description or prediction are

Fig. 6.8.
Separation of Function: Machine.

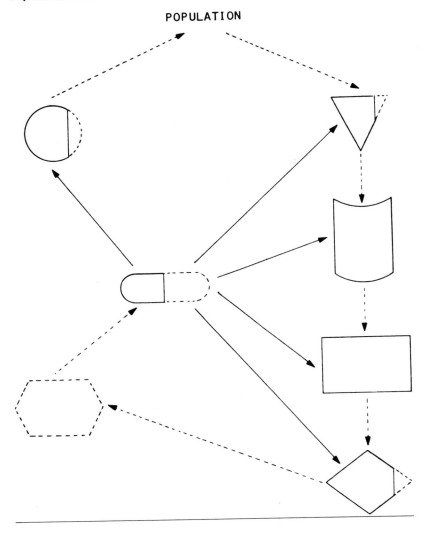

POPULATION

1. There is a *difference* between measurements.
2. Objects A and B can be *classified* appropriately.
3. These findings are *reproducible*.

This information is used by the human to interpret, to modify, and to reconstruct a body of knowledge. This, in turn, leads to redefinition of the problem to be studied as well as the criteria for studying it. The process is cyclical. The specific associations to a symbol may change, depending on

Fig. 6.9.
The Scientific Method.

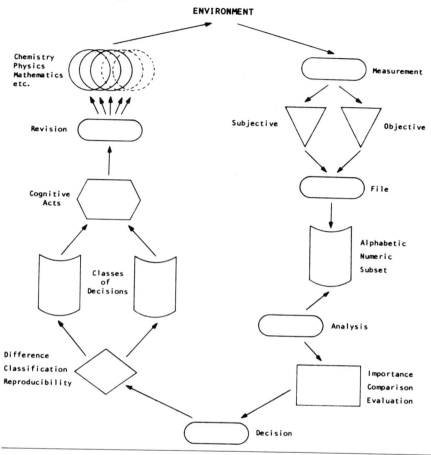

changes in content of other symbols. This property is derived primarily from the process performed in the *cognitive* function. Here an observation, procedure, or result is modified to fit into the structure. The existing body of knowledge is also transformed when it accepts the new element.

Summary
This chapter outlined means by which the interactions between the investigative-care team and the patients can be depicted in terms of six functions:

1. contact (communication)
2. measurement
3. file (storage and retrieval)
4. analysis

5. decision-making
6. cognitive effort (criteria, etc.)

These combined functions form a "molecule" of behavioral activity descriptive of one aspect of a process or of an entire process. The graphic profile of these functions allows translation to a critical analysis using mathematical models or simulation techniques. These results, in turn, permit finer specification of procedures used.

The analysis of functions integrates the questions posed in clinical research design with clinical decision analysis of care.

Chapter 7

Allocation and Monitoring

Introduction

The class of studies designed to answer medical questions are called medical trials. The study may deal with diagnostic, therapeutic, or surveillance issues. The environment in which the study is conducted may vary from a single clinic or laboratory to a geographically dispersed consortium of institutions. The participating disciplines may vary from one to many.

The importance of the investigative process is reflected in repeated appeals to apply the methodology to daily patient management. For example, Pickering (1949) suggested that

Therapeutics is the branch of medicine that, by its very nature, should be experimental. . . . Had it been done we should have gained a very precise knowledge of the place of individual methods of therapy in disease, and our efficiency as doctors would have been enormously enhanced.

Fredrickson (1968) introduced a discussion of the multi-institutional, cooperative clinical trial (the field trial) as follows:

The first recorded field trial took place many years ago in the Garden of Eden. The experimental protocol had received inadequate prior consideration, the population sample was too small, the study consumed too large a fraction of the gross national product at the time, and the results, while considered by some to be unequivocal, have generally been felt to have been overinterpreted.

The potential interrelationships in the study may be simply depicted, as shown in Figure 7.1. The triad of factors begins with the characteristics of the host. In human studies, attributes such as age, sex, socio-economic status, personality factors, etc., have been used to select individuals for

Fig. 7.1.
Relationships in Therapeutics.

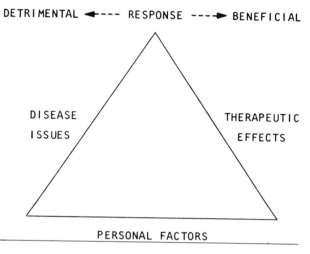

DETRIMENTAL ◄--- RESPONSE ---► BENEFICIAL

DISEASE
ISSUES

THERAPEUTIC
EFFECTS

PERSONAL FACTORS

investigation of the relationship between disease and therapy. There have
been numerous examples of incorrect interpretations of therapy effects.
Frequently, the patients' personal factors were found to be of greater importance in predicting outcome than the therapy used. Statistical assignment
techniques have been developed to minimize the influence of these personal
factors. While known factors can be minimized using various means, the
unknown factors can be minimized only by using the statistical methods.
The inability to document the fact that unknown factors have been balanced
between the treatment groups has led to controversy among investigators
in terms of the effectiveness of the methods in accomplishing the intended
minimization.

Two components of human studies, allocation and monitoring of
responses, will be discussed in some detail in this chapter.

A critical issue in design is the distinction between

1. identification of a therapy which is *best* for a *group,* and
2. identification of a therapy which is *best* for an *individual.*

The therapy will be considered *best* for individuals and for groups when
the therapy completely overwhelms the disease (ignoring differences in
the humans); when the humans respond to the therapy in a single unique
way (despite differences in the disease); or when there are no variations in
the humans or in the disease. In this latter situation, the genetic background
and the phenotypic representations are singular. In other situations, the
therapy may be best for either the group or the patient.

Much of the problem in recognition of effective therapy stems from the emphasis placed on the individual dimensions of the triad. As implied in Figure 7.1, by choosing the interaction between disease and the individual as the most pertinent, the *ethical* emphasis would be toward a judgmental (non-equal probabilities) selection of therapy; that is, the physicians choose the treatment *best* for the patient. The use of random selection (equal probabilities) can be accepted as ethical when the disease-personal relationships are not *clearly* known. In this situation, the therapy may be *best* for the group, the individual, or for neither.

The identification of therapeutic approaches which match the disease-personal variations may represent an interim state. The available therapies may be insufficient to overwhelm differences between individuals. This was the status in bacterial pneumonias prior to introduction of antibiotics. If the investigator believes that the therapy must have a global beneficial effect and it cannot accomplish this, then the conclusion will be "no benefit" to the *group*, even though there are individuals who show the desired outcome.

As an example, the use of coronary bypass surgery has been discussed as part of a series entitled *Controversies in Cardiology.* C. R. Conti (1978) summarized the findings with:

Coronary bypass surgery can be performed with a low rate of morbidity and mortality and can successfully reduce or eliminate symptomatic angina pectoris. However, it is not yet clear whether the procedure prolongs life. A definitive answer to this question requires long-term prospective data on patients undergoing surgical or medical therapy who are comparable in degree of ventricular impairment, severity of symptoms and type and extent of coronary artery disease.

J. W. Hurst and his colleagues (1978) summarized the findings as follows:

Four methods, none perfect, have been used to compare the results of such surgery with the results of medical therapy . . . It is therefore time to analyze the available data in light of the treacherousness of the disease and to determine if a clear trend is evident . . . properly performed coronary bypass surgery will increase coronary blood flow and relieve angina pectoris in 90 percent of patients; total relief of angina can be expected in 60 percent and partial relief in 30 percent. Compared with modern medical therapy, properly performed coronary bypass surgery appears to prolong the life of patients who have obstruction of the left main coronary artery or triple or double vessel disease. There is not adequate evidence to state that the procedure will prolong the life of patients with single vessel obstruction.

The designs used in the studies reviewed by Hurst et al. were

1. *Retrospective matched studies. This method entails creating a study plan (protocol) and applying it to previously observed patients. . . .*

2. *Prospective matched studies. This method entails creating a study plan (protocol) and entering patients into the study as they are observed. Some patients will be entered into a surgical and some into a medical group. . . .*

3. *Prospective randomized study. Theoretically, this should be the best method of performing clinical trials. Practically, it often is not. . . .*

4. *Comparison of study groups with life tables. The Department of Health, Education, and Welfare has generated life tables that permit one to estimate the yearly survival rate of persons living in the United States. Various insurance companies have made similar tables. . . .*

These designs illustrate the range available to investigate a therapeutic relationship. The two issues repeatedly raised are the allocation of therapy and the use of comparison groups. The latter incorporates the processes and problems in monitoring responses.

Allocation
Inherent in the statistical methods used in allocation of study subjects to experimental groups is the need to categorize the individual as a member of a group included in the study. That is, when there is choice of therapy, the study subjects available for receipt of these choices should be as comparable as possible at the outset. With this *matching* accomplished, final assignment should employ random methods.

A recent study by Gardner and Barker (1975) reported results in the assignment of individuals to one of two groups. The problem of assignment rapidly became impossible as the number of variates increased. They used nine questions, each representing a symptom. The answers expected were "absent" or "present." With nine dichotomous variates, there are 2^9 possible outcomes. However, the assignment process complicates this usual outcome problem by creating the classes:

1. *predicted* as disease
2. *not predicted* as disease.

Instead of 2^9 outcomes, there are 2^{2^9} or 2^{512} divisions. The number of possibilities can be reduced by developing a classification rule which collapses divisions.

The Bayes theorem should be the most effective device for calculating probabilities needed for assignment information. As was discussed in Chapter 2, the probability of disease i, given the symptoms X, is $P(D_i|X)$,

Table 7.1
Methods for Assignment of an Individual to One of Two Exclusive Groups

Method	Percent Patients Assigned as "Disease"	
	First Sample	**Second Sample**
Full Multinomial	70	15

$$\hat{P}(X|D_i) = n_i(X)/n_{i,}$$

$n_i(X)$ = number with response vector X
in sample n_i from i^{th} population.
$2^P - 1$ parameters are estimated.

Independence	70	63

$$\hat{P}(x_j = 1|D_i) = \sum_{S_j} n_i(X)/n_i$$

where S_j is the set of responses
X which have $x_j = 1$.

$$\hat{P}(X|D_i) = \prod_{j=1}^{P} \hat{P}(x_j = 1|D_i)^{x_j} \{1 - \hat{P}(x_j = 1|D_i)^{1-x_j}\}$$

Nearest Neighbor	70	71

$$\lambda(X) = \left\{\sum_{S_j} n_1(X_i)/n_1\right\} / \left\{\sum_{S_j} n_0(X_i)/n_0\right\}$$

S_j is the set of response vectors X_i and
$(X - X_i)'(X - X_i) \leqslant r$. (Order 2)

Combination of Symptoms	70	56

$$\lambda(c) = \left\{\sum_{S_j} n_1(x_i)/n_1\right\} / \left\{\sum_{S_j} n_0(X_i)/n_0\right\}$$

where S_j is the set of response vectors X_j
such that $X_j'c = r$. New vectors, c, have
r ones and $(p - r)$ zeros to denote the $\binom{P}{r}$
possible combinations of r symptoms
present, $r = 1 \ldots p$.

Stepwise Procedures	70	50

1. Choose variate which alone has
   maximum information divergence;

2. Split samples from each population
   into two cells using this variate;

3. Find next variate which divides each
   cell into best divergent pair;

4. Continue process until no further selection.

Table 7.1 *Cont*
Methods for Assignment of an Individual to One of Two Exclusive Groups

Method	Percent Patients Assigned as "Disease"	
	First Sample	Second Sample
Linear Discriminant Function	70	60

$$\log_e \lambda\,(X) = \{X - \tfrac{1}{2}\,(\mu_1 + \mu_0)\}\textstyle\sum^{-1}(\mu_1 - \mu_0)$$

μ_1 and μ_0 are the population means.
$\sum$ represents identical dispersion matrices.

Method		
Multiple Logistic Function	70	63

$$\text{logit } P(D_1|X) = \text{logit } \{1 - P(D_0|X)\}$$
$$= (1,X')\beta$$

where logit $y = \log_e \{y/(1-y)\}$
and $\beta' = (\beta_0, \beta_1 \ldots \beta_p)$ is the
vector of logistic coefficients.

Method		
Number of Symptoms	70	67

$$\hat{\lambda}(X) = \left\{\sum_{S_j} n_1(X_j)/n_1\right\} \Big/ \left\{\sum_{S_j} n_0(X_j)/n_0\right\}$$

where S_j is the set of response vectors X_j,
$X_j'L = k$ and L is the (p $\times$ 1)
unit vector.

where $X = (x_1 \ldots x_p)$ is the vector of observations. Each x_j is either 0 or 1 and corresponds to the absence or presence of the jth symptom, $j = 1, 2, \ldots p$. The disease states, D_i, are not disease ($i = 0$) and disease ($i = 1$). The likelihood ratio is $\lambda(X) = P(X|D_1)/P(X|D_0)$. This allocates the individual to D_1 if $\lambda(X) > A$ and otherwise to D_0. $A = P(D_0)/P(D_1)$.

The methods used by Gardner and Barker are shown in Table 7.1. The full multinomial method failed with the second set of independent data but all of the assignment methods worked in the original sample. As is common practice, the first data set was used to develop the classification values. The surprising result was that the sum of positive symptoms performed well in the second, independent data sample. As discussed earlier, this sum ignores the ranking of the variates' importance in diagnosis.

Given the assignment of the individual to a study group, the allocation of therapy may be based on a variety of strategies.

Simple Random Assignment
This method for two treatments matches the sequence of randomly generated even and odd numbers with the assignment of one of two therapies. If three therapeutic regimens are involved, the sequence of random numbers is partitioned into *aliases* for each of the three therapies. This may be

accomplished using rules such as: therapy 1—1, 2, 3; therapy 2—4, 5, 6; therapy 3—7, 8, 9. The number zero would be ignored.

The occurrence of random digits satisfies the criteria of both equal frequency and independence. The assumption that random assignment insures equal frequencies for both known and unknown attributes in the treatment groups is not necessarily satisfied. Imbalances in characteristics can occur, when patients are not all available at one time but are entered sequentially. Matching random numbers, treatment assignments, and unknown patient attributes can and does result in assignment schemes which do not protect against the sources of confounding. This technical problem had led to the use of blocking and stratification to improve random assignment balances.

Blocked Random Assignment
This scheme is used to force balance of the treatment groups after a fixed number of random assignments. As an example, consider three treatment groups with balancing to be accomplished for each group of six patients entered sequentially. The process is illustrated in Table 7.2. As shown, random assignments to any treatment group cannot exceed two in every set of six. This is shown by the columns "random" and "nonrandom." Nonrandom are forced assignments for balancing. The assignment rule is shown at the bottom of the table. The observed sequence is given at the bottom, as well as in the column labeled "random."

Stratified Random Assignment
In this scheme, the random assignment takes place within each stratum or subgroup of study subjects. The strata are defined in terms of presenting factors representing differing anticipated responses to therapy, so that balancing of the treatments *must* be performed in order to interpret the results. Either of the two previously discussed schemes could be applied to the individual strata.

The problem with this scheme is that the uneven entry sequence throws assignments of therapy off balance. The disproportionate entry gives rise to potentially large imbalances in comparisons of overall treatment effects. This is particularly cogent, in that stratification may have been used to minimize the effects of those entry variates rather than to establish comparisons within each subgroup. Current practice does not recommend this method because of the possible imbalances and because there are other models better adapted to this problem.

Dynamic Allocation
With these schemes, treatment assignments are performed within strata until it becomes necessary to force assignment in order to balance the number assigned to each treatment group overall.

Table 7.2
Example of Blocked Random Assignments

Sequence Number	Random*	Nonrandom	Assigned Group
1	3	—	1
2	7	—	3
3	9	—	3
4	1	—	1
5	—	X	2
6	—	X	2
7	1	—	1
8	4	—	2
9	3	—	1
10	8	—	3
11	6	—	2
12	—	X	3
13	5	—	2
14	9	—	3
15	1	—	1
16	2	—	1
17	8	—	3
18	—	X	2
.	.	.	.
.	.	.	.

*Random Rule and Sequence: 1 = 1, 2, 3; 2 = 4, 5, 6; 3 = 7, 8, 9;
3, 7, 9, 1, 1, 4, 3, 8, 6, 5, 9, 1, 2, 8, ②, 7, 9, 0, 2, 1

A relatively simple mechanism for attempting manual control of an adaptive process is shown in Table 7.3. As seen, two treatments are considered in each of two strata. The three columns shown indicate the operation of random and forced assignment. Column A represents those assigned to one treatment; column B represents those assigned to another. The middle column represents the adjustment process. Beginning in the middle, the possible paths are indicated by arrows. It is impossible to have more than two consecutive assignments to either A or B. The opposite treatment is forced into operation avoiding these runs. This scheme allows one to consider the past assignments within the stratum and provide a close balance overall.

Summing the actual assignments to A gives a total of nine patients. The

Table 7.3
Adaptive Assignment

	Stratum 1				Stratum 2		
Patient ID	**A**	**X**	**B**	**Patient ID**	**A**	**X**	**B**
1	←———			2		———→	
4	———→			3		←———	
5		———→		6	←———		
7		←———		8	———→		
11		———→		9			———→
12		←———		10			←———
13	←———			14		———→	
15	———→			16		←———	
17	←———			18		———→	
.				.			
.				.			
.				.			

assignments to B also total nine patients. Within Stratum 1, the assignments were: 5 to A, 4 to B. Within Stratum 2, they were: 4 to A, 5 to B.

Conditional Allocation

A number of schemes involve using the present findings in assigning treatment to the next individual or group of individuals. These plans, being conditional on the presently "best" therapy, reduce objections to random assignment schemes. Patients are assigned at random only until a "better" rule is available. That rule is based on the better therapy. The rule is changed either to a random one or to alternate therapy when a failure is observed with the present assignment scheme.

A simple schema for these plans is given in Table 7.4. As seen, the first assignment uses random allocation. The result is observed and is a "success." The next patient then receives the same therapy. When the result is a "failure," the next patient then receives the other therapy (B). The result is success. Random assignment is used when there is no better rule to follow. This is shown with patients 4, 5, and 6. Patient number 4 was a failure on B; patient 5 was a failure on A; choose therapy for patient 6 using random assignment.

Sequential Allocation

The emphasis in these strategies is on recognition of the difference between therapy regimens rather than on assignments. Indeed, the assignments can include simple random or blocked random plans. The major advan-

Table 7.4
Assignments Using a Combination of Random Methods and Results from Preceding Patients

Patient ID	Choose A	B
	(at random)	
1	S	
2	F	
3		S
4		F
5	F	
	(at random)	
6		F
7	S	
8	F	
9		S
10		S
11		S
12		S
13		F
14	F	
15		S
16		S
etc.		

NOTE: S = Success; F = Failure.

tage is that analysis can be continuous with the recognition of a therapeutic advantage at the earliest moment. The sample size tends to be smaller than for nonsequential designs.

Usual Schemes
Of the plans discussed, the most frequent schemes are simple and blocked randomization. Another frequently used strategy is the stratified random assignment. These plans involve fixed sample sizes and are not designed to guard against the probabilistic consequence of multiple interim analyses. Certainly, the schemes do not include the flexibility offered by either the sequential or conditional assignment plans.

In the most recent review of design and analysis for clinical trials, the recommendation was for simple or blocked randomization. The feeling was that the available analytical techniques could account for the potential front-end differences while assessing treatment effects.

Monitoring Conduct and Performance

Implicit in some allocation schemes and explicit in others is concern about assigning patients to less effective therapy. This concern motivates patient monitoring so that events of interest can be readily determined. The data capture process is an integral part of patient management. Data recording and analysis are formalized information processing components in the research program. While a variety of analytical models may be used, the decision-making portion is a component of monitoring.

It has been known for some time that the multiple use of a conventional test rule of the form

$$P \, (\text{Statistic} > \text{Critical Value}) \leqslant \alpha,$$

where α is the defined probability area from the critical value to plus infinity, can lead to an actual probability much greater than α. This phenomenon is shown in Table 7.5. The results reflect multiple independent testing. Note

Table 7.5
Multiple Testing and Resulting Probability

Number of Tests	Actual Level of Significance	
	0.05	0.01
1	0.05	0.01
2	0.10	0.02
3	0.14	0.03
4	0.19	0.04
5	0.23	0.05
6	0.26	0.06
7	0.30	0.07
8	0.34	0.08
9	0.37	0.09
10	0.40	0.10
11	0.43	0.10
12	0.46	0.11
13	0.49	0.12
14	0.51	0.13
15	0.54	0.14

that the .01 level of significance, if more stringent for a single test, changes less for multiple tests. The monitoring process must take into account both the distortion from multiple testing and the need to determine consistent priorities for therapeutic effects.

Problems of assessing therapy in relationship to conflicting adverse endpoints have been observed in national studies employing data safety and monitoring committees. For example, the Coronary Drug Project faced difficulties in deciding to stop a therapy. Estrogen and dextrothyroxin regimens were terminated earlier than anticipated because of adverse effects. The high dose estrogen regimen was stopped after observing an increased number of non-fatal myocardial infarctions and an increased number of pulmonary embolic episodes. The other regimen was stopped after observation of an association between initial arrhythmia and later non-fatal myocardial infarction.

These adverse effects, being non-fatal, were part of the event set considered important primarily for final analysis. However, for monitoring, the single significant effect was death. Therapies were to be terminated if there were a significant number of deaths. The dilemma faced by the Data Safety Monitoring Committee was when non-fatal events could be considered as significant as fatal ones.

The other issue was the differential in occurrence of adverse events given front-end factors. This was seen in terms of low-risk and high-risk differences in occurrence of pulmonary emboli and of non-fatal myocardial infarctions with high-dose estrogen therapy. Further, the dextrothyroxin adverse effects were associated with prior occurrence of arrhythmia.

Extrapolating from the Coronary Drug Project, the monitoring process can be characterized as a *series of studies*. The patient moves through these studies as he experiences or avoids occurrence of adverse and beneficial effects. This process is illustrated in Figure 7.2. As seen, the monitoring can be subdivided into immediate, intermediate, and long-term results.

Immediate Effects
The immediate effects represent, in terms of therapy, the selection of appropriate starting doses. In many systems, the therapy is not toxic. Monitoring can then be based on the occurrence of unusual or unanticipated adverse effects. Recognition of an unusual number of toxic events could lead to dose reductions or therapy replacement. In other diseases, the therapy may be anticipated to produce toxicities. Recognition of events may be classified as:

1. those anticipated—no evidence for change
2. those not anticipated—evidence for change.

When establishing these immediate monitoring procedures, definitions are

Fig. 7.2.
Issues in the Monitoring Process.

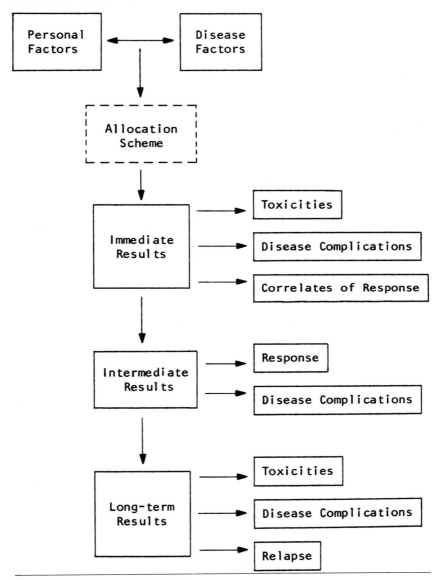

required for the length of the period, the measurements associated with the events, the schedule of data capture, and the number of patients to determine the ''acceptability'' of that portion of the total study. This acceptability testing or quality control is not an incidental function, as the total number of patients are accrued for the primary question raised by the study. As seen in Figure 7.2, each patient must successfully pass through this portion prior to being available for later questions.

Similarly, the immediate occurrence of complications or of precursors of disease regression may be monitored. Complications which are observed immediately following introduction of therapy may be classified as toxicities rather than extensions of the underlying disease process. This distinction may be difficult to define. The monitoring may be structured to recognize complications as a subset of toxicities with appropriate decision criteria.

Precursors of disease regression represent those measures of disease stability and / or improvement which imply rather than document disease regression. The formalization of measurements and analyses in the assessment of this area of beneficial effects may be as important as the recognition of adverse therapeutic events.

Intermediate Effects
The major data capture components deal with documentable disease regression (response) and with disease extension (complication). The intermediate effects phase of a study is comparable to the middle portion of an airplane trip. The excitement of takeoff is past. The landing is a future event. The essential requirements of the middle are to perform the expected and to quickly recognize and react to the unexpected.

Recognition of the onset, the pertinent measurements of this event, and ultimately the duration of response constitute the data capture and analytical elements of response. In an analogous fashion, recognition of extensions of disease involve both data capture and analytical procedures. These are typical patient management processes. As with the other phases, the decision criteria and the associated sample sizes match quality control with information realization.

Long-Term Results
The final phase of the study includes those elements associated with the potentially deteriorating effects of a beneficial therapy. Long-term toxicities represent an undesirable manifestation of beneficial therapy. The primary adverse effect is the loss of disease control. This may be in the form of death or in non-fatal events. As demonstrated by the experience in the Coronary Drug Project, these fatal and non-fatal events establish an ultimate monitor. In that study, the fatal events were to be used to answer the pri-

mary research question of survival benefit. The non-fatal events became critical elements in developing decision criteria regarding continuation of therapies.

Summary

The medical trial process embodies a series of investigative approaches employing diagnostic and therapeutic questions. In addition, the desired information may come from procedures yielding enhanced surveillance without new technology associated with recognition of attributes previously hidden.

The critical issues discussed in design of such trials involve the allocation of patients to defined subgroups (diagnostic and / or therapeutic) and the problems and procedures of monitoring the patients. Monitoring is essential for both patient management and study management.

Chapter 8

Multi-Institutional and Multi-Disciplinary Research

Introduction

Traditionally, a new medical "truth" was established after observing a similar result from each of the "similar," although independent, trials. These studies have been conducted in different geographical locations. The patient population could have been different in minor and major ways. The procedures used could have been similar, and led to studies which usually replicated each other. In contrast, the designs, while appearing similar, could have included significant procedures significantly altering the intended design.

When the results of these independent trials proved to be in agreement with each other, the findings took on even greater importance. These results were interpreted as validation of the effectiveness of the multiple, independent trial format. That is, a new "truth" could be obtained from consensus-supported results when observed in different

1. patient groups
2. geographical, socio-economic, and cultural settings
3. combinations of expertise and motivation in conducting medical trials
4. capabilities and facilities to provide high-quality medical care, both standard and research oriented.

If the consistent study conclusion was taken to mean "truth," what was the interpretation of an inconsistent finding? What would it mean if the independent trials reported equivocal results and equally frequent beneficial or negative findings? Were the procedural differences sufficient to obscure the anticipated findings? If the comparisons failed to demonstrate procedural explanations for conflicting results, were the patient groups representative of the same disease process? More important than a particular disease or trial format, how stable, accurate, and appropriate was the independent trial approach? Did the independence condition offer a better answer than one involving replication using independent patient groups? Were the design and procedures of sufficient dependence to substantiate the claim that the *same study was conducted in each setting?*

The historical development of cooperative clinical studies suggests that the major thrust was to control procedures in the various centers. As significant questions were identified, institutions able to perform the disciplined, reproducible exercise would be selected and organized into a cooperative study. The sample of patients would be the major, possibly the only, source of independence.

Extending a research plan to more than one site is not a simple process. Each new medical environment presents an array of requirements associated with

1. patient screening
2. recruitment capabilities
3. enrollment opportunities
4. treatment facilities (supportive, special, multi-modal)
5. surveillance expertise
6. reporting of findings.

Institutional differences in clinical managment and in clinical research application may be magnified by requirements for contributions from non-clinical and pre-clinical scientists within the institution. That is, the goals envisioned by the clinical scientists will include data viewed by them as integral to the research. The non-clinical and pre-clinical investigators may consider the production of the data to be a service function rather than research. The program planners must adjust their research structure to accommodate the problems and capabilities of each institution to

1. reach compromises so that the multi-disciplinary effort can take place
2. produce questions (clinical and pre-clinical) which create an *innovative, exciting* research program.

Organizational Structure

The committee is an operational entity in the cooperative group structure. Policy is formulated by an executive committee. Performance is monitored by a membership / standards committee. Science is defined by a protocol committee. Administrative matters are conducted by a coordinating committee.

The staff function becomes essential to the operation of such organizations. Were it not for personnel employed to provide the necessary material for review and deliberation by the committee, the respective chairmen would be forced to assume the staff role. Since these individuals and their committee members tend to be geographically dispersed, the requirements placed upon them would be difficult to satisfy.

Coordination in such studies can function smoothly when a group provides

1. a repository for scientific data
2. a capability for analysis of the collected data
3. a facility for preparation of procedural and scientific reports
4. a capacity for fiscal management.

The problems faced in coordinating and managing cooperative research have stimulated development of information processing as a technology. While coordinating centers differ in the mix of methods they use, the multi-institutional nature of the study forces their consideration of a relatively similar set of techniques to be used as the support package. These coordinating centers realistically depict the functions and possiblities of legitimate information processing units.

The coordinating center, in most cooperative studies, is located in a single institution. Accordingly, the disciplines required to provide the services are recruited from that institution. As computer technology has advanced, the necessity for a single location has been reduced. The coordinating center may exist simultaneously in many locations, each having access to the required data and each contributing the necessary expertise. The concept remains of selecting the best persons for the jobs. However, the search may now be restricted only by the breadth of the computer network used for the study. The functions performed are also restricted only by the technological limits of the computer network.

As implied, the group structure is an open one. The opportunity to review the processes used is available to the committees of investigators and to the supporting staff. The research conducted is one which fits a model of continuing public scrutiny. The investigators, willing and able to function effectively in this milieu, appreciate the opportunities provided by this forum. Those who would be threatened by this "goldfish bowl" environment tend to isolate themselves from cooperative research opportunities and to depreciate the importance of the research findings.

The issue is an important one, in that committee-directed research can proceed slowly and awkwardly. It can also represent the contributions of the "best" experts. The rate of progress is dependent, not upon the number of decision makers involved, but rather on the expertise of the information processing staff. The need in committee deliberations is for accurate, available data prepared in a concise and understandable fashion. The alternatives available to the committee should have been identified by the support staff. The associated requirements should have been anticipated. The computer support should be such that simulations and additional analyses are available on request. This information utilization capability is the heart of the effective committee function. When such capabilities are not available, the committee process can appear to be less desirable than the single decision maker.

The contrast is not in the virtues of single versus multiple decision makers or in public versus private decisions. Rather, it is in the availability of data and analyses from which decisions can be made. The cooperative group structure, with its emphasis on the committee process, forces and encourages the development of effective information processing.

Descriptions of the Study
The multi-institutional program must consider different descriptions of the study intended for the various target groups. The descriptions include

1. a prototype of the patient informed consent form
2. a summary protocol for referring physicians
3. a procedures manual for involved investigators and staffs
4. an application containing background, research plan, and justification for a funding agency.

Informed Consent
This document should be a succinct, understandable description of the research. The goals, experimental procedures, risks, and benefits should be elucidated. In addition, the potential participant should be informed about alternate forms of management for his problem. The consent form is evidence of patient involvement in the selection of the experimental approach. He is also required to indicate that he is aware of his freedom to initiate and to discontinue participation without jeopardy.

The virtues and defects in the information transfer associated with consent forms may be the subject of controversy for many years. The problem is primarily an emotional one. The major problem faced by the cooperative study protocol committee is to construct a sample consent form which conforms to the requirements of the Department of Health and Human Services and states the facts of the study in a succinct, concise, and clear fashion. Lastly, the major educational and motivational elements must be included in an acceptable fashion. When these requirements have been satisfied, the prepared form may be modified by each participating institution to meet the specific requirements of the local setting.

Summary Descriptions
The participating investigators frequently represent a large diffuse group of physicians and laboratory scientists who have only mild interest in the proposed study. This latter group is not willing to read through the detailed descriptions of the study but might review a simplified summary highlighting the major themes and procedures in the research.

This summary may be likened in many ways to a sales brochure. The material should be presented artistically. Type size and font should be chosen for appearance and readability. Multi-colored presentations may be considered to be too extreme for the science involved, but summaries have been prepared using matching color combinations for paper and ink.

A second summary format used is the prepared "talk." In this approach, a set of descriptive slides and lecture notes are prepared and distributed to local investigators. The material is used at hospital and association meetings. The length is usually from 10 to 20 minutes. The intention is to present

1. significant findings leading to the study
2. questions to be answered by the study, with appropriate explanations
3. a graphic description of those involved in the study, such as participating institutions, numbers of patients, etc.
4. diagnostic and/or therapeutic issues which could be challenged, with suitable defenses for the approaches taken in the study
5. significance of the study in terms of moneys allocated through previous years, numbers of studies, etc., and
6. mechanisms for patient referral and safeguards for existing physician-patient relationships.

A third summary approach uses the media to appeal directly to the potential patient population. Here the summary may be a set of factual statements including

1. the agency sponsoring the research
2. the number of participating centers
3. eligible persons
4. problem studied
5. addresses and telephone numbers.

These statements could be woven into an interview for television or into a newspaper account.

A fourth approach employs combinations of these. For example, a program might be developed for a national association meeting. Scientific presentations might be followed by discussions focused on the issues of group formation and patient referral. To support the scientific session, brochures may be distributed and posters displayed in the convention area.

Procedures Manuals
The purpose of this description is to state the details of each step of the study. The laboratory procedures of special research studies may or may not be included but the essential materials (specimens, timing, etc.) required to perform the laboratory analysis must be included if other branches of the study team participate in preparing or obtaining them.

The procedures manual is typically considered to be an elaboration of the research plan (or protocol). However, the scientific rationale for the study is not necessarily included nor are the various references used in the study. The required elements are

1. screening procedures
2. recruitment procedures
3. enrollment procedures
4. assignment to therapy
5. surveillance schedule and procedures
6. therapy modification rules
7. patient stopping rules
8. special studies procedures
9. reporting procedures.

These categories are not foreign to those in the research plan. The intention is to provide specific and detailed instructions for the staff who perform the tasks rather than to inform outside reviewers. As such, the manual should be structured to serve the needs of those who will use it.

A critical component in the manual is the detailed, "all-inclusive" subject index and glossary of terms. The user *must* be able to reach the desired procedure by *any* relevant word or associated phrase route. A major effort in definition and cross-indexing of terms is necessary to reduce error in patient processing. There is a psychological advantage as well, in that the user can quickly identify this attention to detail and respond in kind.

In addition to the required elements in the procedure, a rationale for the procedure should be provided, even if it seems obvious. However, the obvious rationale should be used in a secondary way and a primary one should emphasize a different aspect. This idea might be clarified by considering the requirement for personal identification. While there are obvious reasons for identifying the patient, the subject could be described through a combination of elements. For example, consider the following list and identify the minimal set to uniquely identify the individual:

1. name
2. address
3. telephone number
4. age
5. date of birth
6. sex
7. race
8. mother's maiden name
9. social security number.

The obvious answer is the social security number. If that is removed from the list, the subset is . . . .

The intention of the procedural description is to reduce error. In addition, the explanations should motivate compliance through understanding of the process and the reasons for it. Motivation should also come from the realization that the study is an important one requiring the individual's best effort.

Another benefit provided by the procedures manual is the opportunity to "test" the process. By identifying the flow of steps and by detailing their rationale and procedures, the process can be critically reviewed. This simulation of the study may be compared with that from the construction of data management and computer support procedures. If the patient management associated study processes "match" the data management mechanisms, the study should be ready for preliminary trial in selected clinics. These should be undertaken to validate the descriptions in the procedural manual and to document the efficacy of the flow.

Funding Agency Applications
These study descriptions are, in some ways, the most difficult to develop. The group which will review and judge the application knows the field, the current research efforts, and the individuals making successful contributions. The application should be written with respect for this preexisting expertise.

Proposed research designed to support current trends and findings has little appeal unless it can be shown that there are possibilities in employing existing leads. A "me too" research project has little charm. A "next step" in a definite direction creates more interest.

Research designed to refute existing beliefs also has little appeal. This approach will be unrewarding if the motivation is simply to show that the rest of the workers in a field are wrong. Where truth is unknown, definitions of "right" or "wrong" may be based on majority opinion. An alternate proposal can receive support if it shows that another interpretation of existing "facts" could be a "next step" study.

The intention is not to mock the review process nor to manipulate it but to emphasize that projects which take advantage of existing findings and proceed in a critically accepted direction have a better chance of being funded.

The multi-institutional and multi-disciplinary project may be less subject to the pressures of creating "me too" research than single institution-based programs. However, a major reason for the multi-institutional approach may be to accrue sufficient numbers of patients. Elements of duplication could creep in through the guise of a "final demonstration of a basic truth." Such finality is rarely rewarded.

In preparing the application for funding, the investigators must come to grips with the relevance of their proposed work. A critical review must answer the question: "Is it 'worth' the money requested?" A second question must be answered by each participating investigator: "Is the proposed research 'worth' the time and energy I must devote to it?" These questions and their answers are related directly to the thrust of the research. If the research duplicates previous work, the answers are negative; if it is innovative, the answers are positive. If the work is not quite at either extreme, the investigators have not properly designed the research and are not ready to request funding.

Feasibility Analyses

The multi-institutional study is subjected to more reviewers than other research study forms. One reason for scrutiny is that each of the participants critically evaluates the study, its potential, and its value. Another reason is the amount of money allocated. The larger the amount, the more critical the review. As a result of these various inspections, this organizational format includes a formalized emphasis on feasibility assessments.

States and Transitions

One approach to feasibility analysis is to depict the patients' entry characteristics, their changed characteristics, and their final status. One simple example of the states would be

State	Condition
1	Normal Health Status
2	Ill
3	Dead

States may be defined by such specific variates as:

State	Age	Variates Rx 1	Rx 2	Status
1	Young	No	No	Well
2	Young	Yes	No	At Risk
3	Young	Yes	Yes	Ill
4	Young	No	No	Dead
.	.	.	.	.
.	.	.	.	.
.	.	.	.	.

As seen, varying the values of the variates provides a multi-factor description of the individual which may be summarized by the label: State 1, State 2, ... Accordingly, states are defined by the values of associated variates. In testing feasibility issues, an obvious question is, "Do the variates define states? If so, how effective (i.e., how unique) is the classification?" Issues of this type were considered in Chapter 7 in relation to the study by Gardner and Barker.

Inherent in all medical studies is the question of effectiveness (in terms of the variates and classification rule used) of assignment to study groups. These assignment rules, in contrast to therapy allocation methods, are used to define the entry, intermediate, and final states for each patient. The flow process is as cogent and sound as the state classification rules.

Given defined states, the recognition of transition implies a change in the associated variates. A second form of feasibility assessment is to determine this functional change. Of particular importance is the question: "Are there variates not included in the state definition which changed in a more dramatic fashion than did those variates which define the states and transitions among them?"

Consider the description of states in acute lymphocytic leukemia shown in Figure 8.1. Patients may be defined as "low" risk to death, "moderate" risk, or "high" risk based on combinations of age and WBC values. The entry states show the low, moderate, and high risk definitions. None of these variates is a significant predictor of remission induction success. Pretreatment values of total white blood cell count and age are related to survival duration in a decreasing fashion during the first three years following induction. After three years of continuous remission, the pretreatment values are no longer related to survival duration. First remission failure is strongly related to survival duration, no matter when it occurs.

Transitions are also illustrated in Table 8.1 which shows the changes that may be observed. The columns depict the influence of a covariate on the transition. Those covariates which might be significantly related to the transition are labeled as "S" and those which might be nonsignificant are labeled as "NS." Unknowns are indicated by "?."

Studies are presently under way which may assist in clarifying complex interrelationships such as those shown in the figure and table. Two outcomes are desirable in constructing interpretations. These are

1.   The influence of covariates on transitions should be possible when considering each transition separately.
2.   Only covariates with significant effects on each transition should be involved in predicting initial to final state transitions.

The first preferred outcome would allow exploration of selected transitions using various statistical approaches to determine significant covariates. The second outcome chooses as the "front to end" subset that set

Fig. 8.1.
States in Acute Lymphoblastic Leukemia.

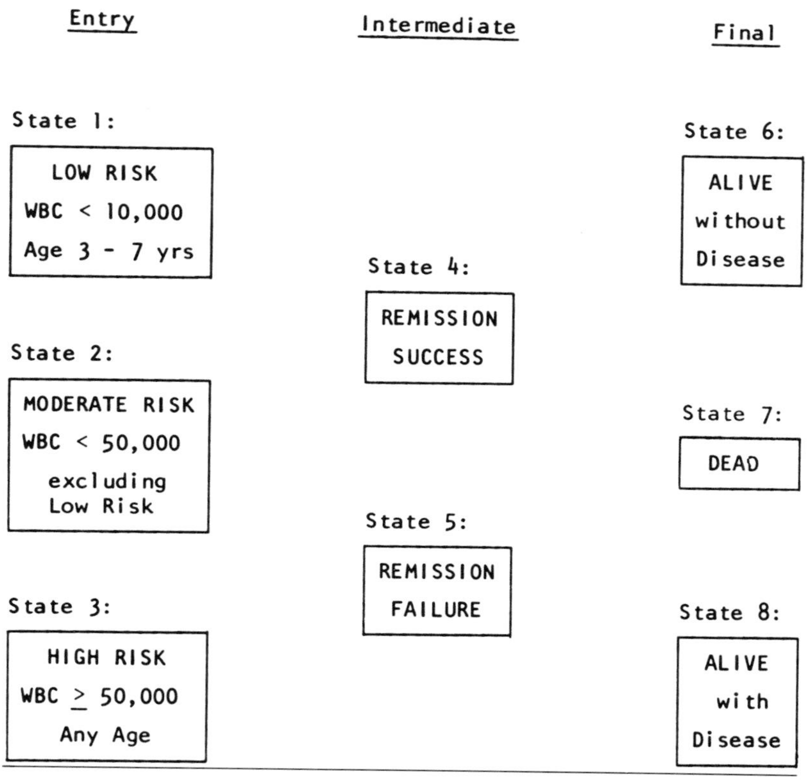

<u>Entry</u>   Intermediate   Final

State 1:   State 6:

┌─────────────────┐   ┌──────────┐
│ LOW RISK   │   │ ALIVE   │
│ WBC < 10,000   │   │ without │
│ Age 3 - 7 yrs   │   State 4:   │ Disease │
└─────────────────┘   ┌─────────────┐   └──────────┘
                          │ REMISSION   │
State 2:   │ SUCCESS   │
                          └─────────────┘
┌─────────────────┐   State 7:
│ MODERATE RISK   │   ┌──────────┐
│ WBC < 50,000   │   │ DEAD   │
│   excluding   │   └──────────┘
│   Low Risk   │   State 5:
└─────────────────┘   ┌─────────────┐
                          │ REMISSION   │
State 3:   │ FAILURE   │   State 8:
┌─────────────────┐   └─────────────┘   ┌──────────┐
│ HIGH RISK   │   │ ALIVE   │
│ WBC ≥ 50,000   │   │ with   │
│ Any Age   │   │ Disease │
└─────────────────┘   └──────────┘

of covariates which play a significant role in each transition. For example, the transitions leading to State 6 would include

$1 \rightarrow 4, 4 \rightarrow 6$

$2 \rightarrow 4, 4 \rightarrow 6$

$3 \rightarrow 4, 4 \rightarrow 6.$

As seen in Table 8.1, neither white blood count nor age is consistently significant in these transitions. This finding is congruent with interpretations of the disease process; that is, the pretreatment values of white blood count and age appear to be of prognostic value in survival during the first three years after induction. If the patient is in State 6 at three years, the white blood count and age no longer predict future survival duration. Similarly, neither pretreatment, white blood count, nor age are long-term predic-

---

Table 8.1
**Transitions and Covariate Influence in
Acute Lymphoblastic Leukemia**

	Covariates	
Transitions	**WBC**	**Age**
1 → 4*	NS	NS
1 → 5	NS	NS
2 → 4	NS	NS
2 → 5	NS	NS
3 → 4	NS	NS
3 → 5	?	NS
4 → 5	?	NS
4 → 6	S	S
4 → 7	S	S
5 → 7	?	?
5 → 8	?	?
5 → 4†	?	?
6 → 5	?	?

*See Figure 8.1 for states, e.g., 1 → 4 is
low risk to remission success.

†This transition is based on a successful
reinduction program.

---

tors in the transition from remission to failure. Given this failure, there is
an increased risk of death.

Monitoring for Therapeutic Effects
These transition issues have been described without considering therapeutic
effects and questions. In particular, monitoring of therapy should include
transitions from entry to "toxicity" states and then to remission success or
failure states. Therapy associated with an extraordinary frequency of
adverse effects may also be less effective in accomplishing remission.

This monitoring process in terms of feasibility leads to a sample size
question or, rather, a variety of such questions depending on the design
chosen. For example, the simplest form of the design would involve a single
therapy with a defined probability of success; that is, suppose that a drug
is used and that the drug is effective in 20% of the patients treated with
it. A sequential treatment program employing this drug could be monitored
by recording the pattern of failures. If the sequence involved consecutive

failures, how long should it be continued? This question is alternatively stated as "How many patients must be studied before the trial is stopped?" This can be easily calculated, since each patient's outcome is unrelated to any other patient's result. The probability of failure (result) would be given by the binomial equation. This formula is

$$\text{probability of result} = \frac{n!}{r! \, (n-r)!} \, p^r (1-p)^{n-r}$$

where:

r   =   number of successes

n   =   total number studied

p   =   probability of a success (non-failure)

n!   = $n \times (n-1) \times (x-2) \, x \ldots x \, 1$ and $0! \equiv 1$.

The first failure is then:

is $\dfrac{1!}{0! \, 1!} \, p^0 (1-p)^1$

$= 1 \times 1 \times 0.8^1$

$= 0.8$

with:

probability of drug effect = 0.2, and

probability of failure = 0.8.

The probability of observing 14 consecutive failures would be

$$P(0 \text{ success in 14 trials}) = \frac{14!}{0! \, 14!} \, 0.2^0 \times 0.8^{14}$$

$= 1 \times 1 \times 0.044$

$= 0.044.$

Alternatively, the probability of observing one or more successes in 14 consecutive patients would be

$1 - P(0 \text{ success in 14 trials}) = 0.956.$

The first probability describes the Type I error, namely, the chance of rejecting $p \geqslant 0.2$ (when, in fact, $p = 0.2$) due to sampling results yielding an observed value less than 0.2. The second probability represents the

Power of the test for rejecting probabilities of success *less* than p = 0.2 when the true probability is p = 0.2. Accordingly, with 14 consecutive patients, the probability of rejecting p $\geq$ 0.2 is 0.044 with a Power of 0.956 against p < 0.2, given that all 14 patients fail.

If there is one or more response in the first 14 patients an alternative monitoring scheme is required. The purpose is to obtain a better estimate of the proportion responding. The additional patients, it is implied, will stabilize the estimate in some desired direction. It is not clear, in such schemes, if the additional patients are allowed to respond. Suppose, for example, that the first 14 patients included a single response (proportion responding = 1/14 = 0.07). Additional patients are added and all fail. With a total sample of 20 patients, the observed proportion of response is 0.05. Should the sampling process be continued until there is a significantly lower proportion responding than the initial one of 0.07? Alternatively, suppose the 1/14 response is changed to 2/15, 3/16, 4/17, 5/18, 6/19, 7/20, ... When should this sampling process be terminated?

With an assumed true proportion of 0.07 and one observed response, the binomial formula could be used to find the sample size so that the probability of $\leq$ 1 response is approximately 5%. That sample size is 65. Accordingly, a rule based on continued sampling until a proportion was reached which was significantly lower than the intitial 0.07 would require 51 additional patients (a total of 65). The probability of observing > 1 response in a sequential study of the 65 patients would be 94%.

The other rule would be to stop sampling when it became unlikely that the expressed proportion of successes (p = 0.2) could occur, given only 14 patients. With a proportion of 0.2, the probability of $\leq$ 1 response is 0.057 in 21 trials. The probability of > 1 response is 0.943. Accordingly, rejection of 0.2 as the true proportion (Type I error = 0.057) requires an additional seven patients. The final estimate of the proportion responding would be 0.047 (1/21).

Both stopping rules would help reach a decision about the size of responding proportion. However, the number of observations required to reject an observed proportion of 0.07 in favor of an even lower value is too large a price to pay for the information. As seen, rejection of the original estimate (p = *2) required a smaller number of observations *if* the number of responses was restricted to the one seen in the first 14 patients.

The problem of stopping a trial because of too few responses begins to disappear as the number of responses increases. As seen in Table 8.2, a total sample size of 30 patients would be required to decide against the hypothesized proportions of $\leq$ 0.2. With three or more responses, none of the sample sizes shown would be large enough to reject p $\leq$ 0.2. The

Table 8.2
Probabilities of 0, 1, 2, . . . , 5 Responses Given p = 0.2

Sample Size	Responses					
	0	1	2	3	4	5
14	0.044	0.154	0.250	0.250	0.172	0.086
16	0.028	0.113	0.211	0.246	0.200	0.120
18	0.018	0.081	0.172	0.230	0.215	0.151
20	0.012	0.058	0.137	0.205	0.218	0.175
22	0.007	0.041	0.107	0.178	0.211	0.190
30	0.001	0.009	0.034	0.079	0.133	0.172

probability of $\leq$ 3 responses in a sample of size 30 is 0.001 + 0.009 + 0.034 + 0.079 or 0.123. When p = 0.2, the probability of observing > 3 responses in a sample of 30 is then 0.877.

Monitoring for Comparison of Therapies
The monitoring process should focus on each subgroup's behavior separately, even though the study question deals with a contrast in groups. This is particularly important when therapies are involved in the group's definition.

For transitions which compare outcomes, monitoring must take into account differences in behaviors as represented by proportions or distributions. For most monitoring, the patients are described either as experiencing the event (giving rise to the proportion with the event) or in terms of time to the event. In the latter situation, the total groups are tracked through time, with each individual contributing to the shape of the time-related function.

Comparison of these curves may rely on assumptions about the underlying probability distribution (parametric models) or its absence. The latter allows the class of "all" distributions (the non-parametric models). The life table method is a frequently used non-parametric model for analyzing time-related events; its format is shown in Table 8.3.

The individuals are considered at risk to the event until they experience it or are removed for some other reason. This right-handed censoring complicates the analysis, because adjustments are arbitrary at best. Appeal to their efficacy is done by showing the proper behavior of the model when there is *no censoring*. Note that there is no intermediate censoring in Table 8.3. Those who did not experience the event leave the analysis after the sixth time interval.

Table 8.3
Life Table Computations

Interval	Number at Risk (L)	Number with Event	q	p	$\dfrac{q}{pL}$	P	Q
1	100	2	0.02	0.98	0.0002	0.98	0.02
2	98	4	0.04	0.96	0.0004	0.94	0.06
3	94	10	0.11	0.89	0.0013	0.84	0.16
4	84	8	0.10	0.90	0.0013	0.76	0.24
5	76	20	0.26	0.74	0.0046	0.56	0.44
6	56	14	0.25	0.75	0.0060	0.42	0.58
.	.	.	.	.	.	.	.
.	.	.	.	.	.	.	.
.	.	.	.	.	.	.	.

NOTE: q = Number with event / number at risk

p = 1 − q

P = Πp

Q = 1 − P

The cumulative survival probability curve is used to evaluate the group's behavior and to compare with other groups. This cumulative probability, P, may be treated as the proportion in a binomial problem. For life table calculations, according to Greenwood, the variance of P is:

$$\text{Var } (P_i) = P_i^2 \sum \frac{q_i}{p_i L_i}.$$

The statistic p_i is the estimated probability of survival during the time interval i; $q_i = 1 - p_i$; and L_i is the number at risk during the interval. P_i is the estimated cumulative probability through interval i.

If this description of the variance of P is compared with the binomial variance formula, with P and $1 - P = Q$, the binomial N becomes the "effective" sample size from the life table. This is:

$$N = \frac{Q}{P \sum \frac{q_i}{p_i L_i}},$$

the number of non-censored patients who would be followed from entry through the risk period and give a standard error equivalent to a larger number of persons with censoring.

The value of N from Table 8.3 (with no censoring) would be

$$N = \frac{Q_6}{P_6 \sum_{i=1}^{6} q_i/p_iL_i}.$$

The sum is $0.0002 + 0.0004 + \ldots + 0.0046 + 0.0060$ or 0.0138. $Q_6 = 0.58$, and P_6 is 0.42. n is then $0.58/0.42(0.0138) = 100$, the number without censoring at risk at the outset, giving the standard error observed at the sixth time period. This number, of course, agrees with the entry number in Table 8.3, as this table was computed without censored data.

In comparing cumulative survival proportions at a preselected time, the binomial again may be used. The equation is, with z as a normal deviate:

$$z = \frac{P_1 - P_2}{\sqrt{\dfrac{P_1(1 - P_1)}{N_1} + \dfrac{P_2(1 - P_2)}{N_2}}}.$$

This estimate of difference is useful in establishing monitoring rules, since a time can be identified in advance. Suppose it is known that the patients pass through a critical point in the disease after three months of therapy. The individual survival curves would be used to compute the effective sample sizes and survival probabilities for comparison in the above equation. The experience would be compared at the end of the third month. The issues and calculations described in this monitoring process are considerably different from an analysis based on the comparison of the biggest observed difference in Ps. Clearly, this analysis is prejudiced in data points used and will provide neither clinical nor probabilistic interpretation.

Monitoring the Primary Study
The final sample size-feasibility issue involves the models and choice of a sample size to test the *main* study question. Even though this was the stated purpose of the study, the ability to analyze the data will come later in time than those intermediate quality control and monitoring questions already considered. The stated purpose may never be analyzed if the study is stopped because of early results. The choice of model for analysis, the earliest time to apply the model, and the smallest number of completed patient experiences required for this first attempt to answer the main question are issues within the general area of feasibility. The optimum time to apply the model and the associated sample size also are feasibility issues.

A contrasting approach to assessing study feasibility ignores all intermediate analyses. The focus would be on entry factors and their relationship to outcome as defined by the study purpose. Time of inititation of the analysis may not be considered. If it is, the final sample size should be adjusted for multiple applications of the models through time. In this approach, the essential features are the statistical model, the values of the decision error probabilities, and the hypothesized study findings. The latter present the investigator's estimate of the results in terms of statistical parameters. The error probabilities are selected to control the sample size by specifying the magnitudes of the potential erroneous decisions.

The Type I error describes the probability of rejecting a true hypothesis. The Type II error describes the probability of accepting a false hypothesis. The statistical model may be used to integrate the statistical and decision parameters and to produce a sample size estimate.

These machinations will be performed even when the various intermediate analyses are considered in addition to the main one. The distinction lies in the possible adjustment of the sample size to include sufficient observations for the many analyses required. The adjustment may not be sizable if the study process accommodates to the sequential flow of the patients from entry through intermediate states to the final ones. In this situation, the question of sufficient size must be posed for intermediate analyses taking model, decision errors, and hypothesized parameters into account. When these sizes are adequate, the final size also should be sufficient. The adjustment may be substantial if the patients can move between study states in either direction. This process would be observed when patients fluctuate between states of improvement and worsening without transition to defined "final" states. The intermediate period could be lengthy and the total sample size large, in order to contain a sufficient number of patients finally achieving the study outcome.

Summary

The cooperative clinical design blends the essential factors in patient aggregations and environmental influences into a unified and disciplined process of study. By controlling for procedural differences, the hypothesized relationships may be challenged in the different environments and conditions. If the results are consistent, the validity of the relationship is easier to determine and to interpret. If the findings are inconsistent, the explanation would be less dependent on procedure than on faulty hypothesized relationships. Again, interpretation of the findings may deal with the relationships rather than extraneous factors.

The multi-institutional, multi-disciplinary research process is associated with additional benefits. Principal ones are

1. the openness of the research process
2. the pressures to organize and to report study results in a continuing fashion

3.   the opportunities to develop methods for effective capture, utilization, and dissemination of scientific information.

Failure to observe these benefits can be identified with concomitant gaps in information processing.

An essential feature of the cooperative process is the emphasis on planning and on anticipating critical questions and decision-making needs. Monitoring schemes with decision criteria constitute the procedures by which the many investigators, staffs, and reviewers can deal with the disciplined behavior required without jeopardizing the welfare of the patient.

References

Conti, C. Richard. Influence of myocardial revascularization on survival. *Amer. J. Cardiol.* 42:330–332, 1978.

Dudley, H. A. F. Pay-off, heuristics, and pattern recognition in the diagnostic process. *Lancet* 2:723–726, 1968.

Eisenhart, C. The role of a statistical consultant in a research organization. *Proc. Internat. Statis. Conf. III* 308–313, 1947.

Fredrickson, Donald S. The field trial—some thoughts on the indispensable ordeal. *Bull. N. Y. Acad. Med.* 44:985–993, 1968.

Gardner, M. J., and Barker, D. J. P. A case study in techniques of allocation. *Biometrics* 31:931–942, 1975.

Gehan, Edmund A., and Schneiderman, Marvin A. Experimental design of clinical trials. In *Cancer Medicine*, James F. Holland and Emil Frei, III, eds. Philadelphia: Lea & Febiger, 1973.

Hurst, J. Willis; King, Spencer B., III; Logue, R. Bruce; Hatcher, Charles R., Jr.; Jones, Ellis, L.; Craver, Joe M.; Douglas, John S., Jr.; Franch, Robert H.; Dorney, Edward R.; Cobbs, B. Woodfin, Jr.; Robinson, Paul H.; Clements, Stephen D., Jr.; Kaplan, Joel A.; and Bradford, James M. Value of coronary bypass surgery—controversies in cardiology: part I. *Amer. J. Cardiol.* 42:308–329, 1978.

Klug, Panpit P.; Lessin, Lawrence S.; and Radice, Peter. Rheological aspects of sickle cell disease. *Arch. Intern. Med.* 133:577–590, 1974.

Konotey-Ahulu, Felix I. D. The sickle cell diseases. *Arch. Intern. Med.* 133:611–619, 1974.

Lessin, Lawrence S., and Jensen, Wallace N., eds. Sickle-cell symposium. *Arch. Intern. Med.* 133:529–713, 1974.

Mainland, Donald. Notes on the planning and evaluation of research, with examples from cardiovascular investigations. *Am. Heart J.* 55:644–655, 824–837, 838–850, 1958.

Peto, R.; Pike, M. C.; Armitage, P.; Breslow, N. E.; Cox, D. R.; Howard, S. V.; Mantel, N.; McPherson, K.; Peto, J.; and Smith, P. G. Design and analysis of randomized clinical trials requiring prolonged observation of each patient. *Br. J. Cancer* 34:585–612, 1976; 35:1–39, 1977.

Pickering, G. W. The place of the experimental method in medicine. *Proc. R. Soc. Med.* 42:229–234, 1949.

Rickles, Frederick R., and O'Leary, Dennis S. Role of coagulation system in pathophysiology of sickle cell disease. *Arch. Intern. Med.* 133:635–641, 1974.

Rogers, D. W.; Vaidya, Shuba; and Serjeant, G. R. Early splenomegaly in homozygous sickle-cell disease—an indicator of susceptibility to infection. *Lancet* 2:963–965, 1978.

Schwartz, William B.; Gorry, G. Anthony; Kassirer, Jerome P.; and Essig, Alvin. Decision analysis and clinical judgment. *Amer. J. Med.* 55:459–472, 1973.

Taylor, Th. R. Clinical decision analysis. *Methods Inf. Med.* 15:216–224, 1976.

Weiner, J. M.; Marmorston, J.; and Meshnik (Wolf), R. *Medical information data analysis system (MIDAS)*. Biostatistics Research Laboratory, Los Angeles, 1972.

Appendix

Information processing is a composite discipline incorporating concepts and methods from the clinical, computer, and statistical sciences. Procedures for the organization and subsequent computer processing of data may be used to illustrate the close interaction between computer and statistical methods. By fitting clinical data into existing computing molds, the investigator can easily obtain analytical results for interpretation and incorporation into existing conceptual structures. Examples of computer and statistical functions are given in this Appendix.

Section 1

Computer Applications

The first applications involve computational methods which do not require prior experience with computers. These programs mimic the operation of desk calculators.

Subsequent examples illustrate a simple method for the collection, organization, and storage of data. Programs providing analyses of such data are introduced.

Data Organization

In preparing for and in performing analyses, the first step is to specify a list of variates. A variate is a general name for a set of numbers. This set may contain whole numbers, fractions, or mixtures. The variate is assigned a name to assist in identifying its relationship with other variates and to indicate its function in the problem considered in the analysis. Examples of variate names are age, sex, time to improvement, white blood count. Each of these names illustrates the characteristics for a variate. For example, the variate AGE may be described either as whole numbers—25, 26, 31, . . . —or as fractions—25.6, 26.1, 31.9, ... Further, the values of numbers should be known when the name of the variate is identified. Thus, human ages are a set of numbers from 0 to 100 (years) or so.

The next step is to obtain the numbers representing the variates from each subject studied. These may be recorded in a variety of ways. Two are shown. The first is a data recording document for a particular subject, listing identifying characteristics and variates.

ID Number _____   Date _____

Name _____

Address _____

_____

Home Tel. # _____   Bus. Tel. # _____

Soc. Sec. # _____   Birth date _____

Sex _____   Height (in) _____   B/P _____

Race _____   Weight (lbs) _____   Pulse_____

Date symptoms first noted: _____

xxxxxx _____

The second is a data summary document for a group of subjects.

ID Number	Sex	Age	Height	Weight	Blood Pressure	Pulse

Note that the data recording document has been transcribed to one line in the data summary document.

To illustrate some immediate computing capabilities which will have long-term usefulness, suppose the data summary document contains the following variates:

ID Number for Subject

Sex (1 = male; 2 = female)

Age (years)

Date Entered Study (displayed as a single number using the format YYMMDD representing the last two digits of the year, two digits for the month, and two digits for the day)

Further, suppose that this information has been obtained for twenty people. The data summary would be as follows:

ID Number	Sex	Age	Date Entered
1	1	30	751201
2	1	25	751203
3	1	40	751215

ID Number	Sex	Age	Date Entered
4	1	53	751226
5	2	37	751231
6	2	44	760109
7	1	16	760122
8	2	69	760124
9	1	72	760212
10	2	33	760220
11	2	28	760302
12	2	30	760310
13	2	54	760328
14	1	26	760407
15	2	19	760410
16	1	52	760412
17	2	43	760421
18	1	66	760515
19	2	19	760601
20	1	48	760615

Note that the use of a sequence number as the person's identification provides the opportunity to know the current total number of subjects studied. Further, entry of the records for new subjects is in date order. Thus, both ID number and date are related in that, as one increases in size, so does the other.

Choosing subgroups of records could be done using either ID number or date. If ID were used and all records with numbers less than 9 were selected, this subgroup would contain those data records for persons who entered before 760201. When two variates agree in terms of information provided as do ID number and date, they are said to *co-vary* (that is, to show variation in numerical value in agreement with each other). Note that the co-variation between these two variates is not perfect. However, one of the two could be used to select a subgroup of records and that subgroup may contain data for other variates which show this agreement with the selecting variate. The variate used to select the subgroup is called a *co-variate* because of this potential agreement with other variates in the record.

Analytical Organization
There are a number of questions which could be posed about the variates shown. For example:

How many males or females have been studied to date?

How many young, middle-aged, elderly persons?

How many persons entered in the first three months?

These "how many" questions are important for a variety of pursuits. If, for example, the answers suggest that very few records exist, some additional questions will not be raised because of insufficient data. Given sufficient data, other questions can be considered.

The "how many" question might be phrased in terms of the question, "What relationship exists between sex and age in persons studied?" To pursue this question, we must first decide what we mean by "age"—that is, young versus not young, old versus not old, etc. Suppose we decide to classify age as:

young = all values less than 40

not young = all values 40 and over.

The relationship between sex and age would then involve selection of those records satisfying one of the criteria:

male *and* young

male *and* not young

female *and* young

female *and* not young.

Each criterion identifies a subgroup of persons. Each subgroup is completely separate and independent of all of the others. These subgroups are represented in the table below by position in the column and row.

	Sex		
Age	**Male**	**Female**	**Total**
Young	4	6	10
Not Young	6	4	10
Total	10	10	20

The male *and* young subgroup includes 4 subjects and is listed in the table in column 1 (male) *and* row 1 (young). All subgroups are shown by title in the next table.

		Column		
		1	**2**	**Total**
Row	**1**	Male and Young	Female and Young	Young
	2	Male and Not Young	Female and Not Young	Not Young
	Total	Male	Female	All Subjects

The rows and columns are defined by numerical intervals which contain the values included in the subgroups. For example, rows are defined by the values 0, 39.9, 100. When these values are taken in pairs, the young are those with values between 0 and 39.9. The limit 39.9 is used to prevent errors in classification; that is, age is recorded to the nearest year. The value for each must be either less or more than 39.9, but cannot be equal to it. It is common to use boundary values extending to one additional digit.

Computer System

The General Electric Mark III Information Network computer system was chosen in order to satisfy particular requirements. These were

1. Ease in Developing New Software.

    The system supports FORTRAN IV at an advanced level. System subroutines provide extensive data, file, and text management capabilities. These subroutines enable the rapid construction of programs which support sophisticated computing.

2. Ease in Managing Data Files.

    The system allows construction of typical file types. Considering the cost-effective management of data, the appropriate file structure to match the study requirements can be chosen and used. Changing from one file structure to another when needs change is easily acccomplished.

3. Availability.

    The system operates on a 24-hour basis with access via teleterminals. Performance can be controlled in terms of "on-line" or batch operations, so that the cost-effective mechanism for execution of required programs can be chosen. This flexibility in use is an important element in meeting changing needs.

4. Equipment Access and Excess.

    The system is designed and functions in a fashion analogous to that expected from a *variable-sized computer,* growing to a sufficiently large size and then shrinking with changing needs. While this concept most readily pertains to storage, it is also applies to interactive versus delayed function. With each mode of operation, the computer system appears to be dedicated to the single user.

Computer Software

The programs in this library are designed to accomplish specific tasks and are structured to maintain significant parameters in common, in order to smooth the transition from one task to the next. The programs operate in an interactive "on-line" fashion and in the delayed "batch" mode. The library is accessed using the code word MIDAS, an acronym for Modular Information Data Analysis System (Weiner 1972).

Functional Descriptions of Programs in the Library

DATA ENTRY

Program Number	Task Performed
2	CONVERT ASCII TO BINARY DATA FILE
50	COMPUTER ASSISTED DATA ENTRY, EDIT, AND STORAGE

FILE MANAGEMENT

Program Number	Task Performed
1	IDENTIFY DATA FILE PARAMETERS
3	INSERT, APPEND, AND LIST RECORDS—DIRECT ACCESS, BINARY FILE
4	CONVERT FROM ONE TYPE OF BINARY FILE TO ANOTHER
5	CONVERT A BINARY TO AN ASCII FILE
8	APPEND BINARY DATA FILES
9	MERGE BINARY DATA FILES
10	SORT A BINARY DATA FILE
11	SELECT SUBSETS OF VARIATES AND / OR RECORDS
45	ORGANIZE DATA FILE FOR QUALITY CONTROL ANALYSES
47	ORGANIZE DATA FILE CONTAINING MULTIPLE RECORDS PER INDIVIDUAL
51	ADD NEW MASTER RECORDS TO A HIERARCHY
52	ADD NEW DEPENDENT RECORDS TO A HIERARCHY
53	REPLACE DEPENDENT RECORDS IN A HIERARCHY
54	DELETE RECORDS FROM A HIERARCHY
56	RESTRUCTURE A HIERARCHICAL FILE
57	RETRIEVE RECORDS FROM A HIERARCHICAL FILE
58	ORGANIZE THE RETRIEVED RECORDS
63	RETRIEVE DATA RECORDS FOR NEW HIERARCHY
80	CONVERT ASCII TO BINARY FILE FOR LONG-TERM STORAGE
81	PURGE FILES
82	EMPTY SEQUENTIAL BINARY FILES

DATA VALUE MANAGEMENT

Program Number	Task Performed
6	COMPARE DATA VALUES FOR VERIFYING ENTERED DATA
7	CHANGE DATA VALUES IN DIRECT ACCESS DATA FILE
12	CONVERT DATES TO SERIAL DAYS AND COMPUTE TIME CHANGES BETWEEN DATES
13	CHANGE SPECIFIED VALUES IN ALL RECORDS
14	TRANSFORM VALUES AND PERFORM SIMPLE CALCULATIONS
59	TRANSFORM VALUES IN HIERARCHICAL DATA STRUCTURES

STATISTICAL COMPUTATIONS

Program Number	Task Performed
17	COMPUTE FREQUENCY TABLES, BAR GRAPHS AND HISTOGRAMS
19	PROVIDE THREE-DIMENSIONAL TABULAR DISPLAYS
22	COMPUTE 2 × 2 CHI-SQUARE TABLES AND TESTS
23	COMPUTE UP TO 10 × 10 CHI-SQUARE TABLES AND TESTS
25	PROVIDE BIVARIATE GRAPHIC DISPLAYS AND COMPUTE LINEAR REGRESSION STATISTICS
26	COMPUTE MEANS AND STANDARD DEVIATIONS
27	COMPUTE CORRELATION COEFFICIENTS
29	COMPUTE GROUP AND PAIRED DIFFERENCE STUDENT T TESTS
32	COMPUTE THE EQUATIONS ASSOCIATED WITH A STEPWISE MULTIPLE LINEAR REGRESSION
35	COMPUTE THE EQUATIONS ASSOCIATED WITH A STEPWISE MULTIPLE LINEAR DISCRIMINANT ANALYSIS
39	COMPUTE MULTI-DIMENSIONAL "LIFE TABLE" TYPE ANALYSES BY SELECTION OF DATA RECORDS CONFORMING TO DEFINED GROUPS
42	COMPUTE MULTIVARIATE "LIFE TABLE" TYPE ANALYSES USING AN EXPONENTIAL REGRESSION EQUATION
43	COMPUTE A NON-LINEAR BINARY REGRESSION EQUATION COMPARING TWO GROUPS
74	COMPUTE BINOMIAL PROBABILITIES FOR DEFINED EVENTS

EQUATION GENERATION

Program Number	Task Performed
36	COMPUTE EQUATION VALUES FROM MULTIPLE LINEAR ANALYSES
75	COMPUTE EQUATION VALUES FROM BIVARIATE LINEAR REGRESSION ANALYSES
78	COMPUTE EQUATION VALUES FROM "LIFE TABLE" TYPE EXPONENTIAL REGRESSION ANALYSES

DISPLAYS

Program Number	Task Performed
15	LIST DATA RECORDS
18	DISPLAY FREQUENCY TABLES, BAR GRAPHS, AND HISTOGRAMS
20	DISPLAY THREE-DIMENSIONAL TABLES
25	DISPLAY BIVARIATE GRAPHS
46	DISPLAY QUALITY CONTROL ANALYSES
60	PROVIDE EDIT MESSAGES IN MULTIPLE RECORD PER SUBJECT ANALYSES

62	DISPLAY DATA FROM MULTIPLE RECORD PER SUBJECT FILES
79	DISPLAY MULTIPLE SIMULATED "LIFE TABLE" TYPE CURVES

MULTIPLE RECORD ANALYSES

Program Number	Task Performed
48	IDENTIFY AND AVERAGE "REPLICATE" RECORDS IN A MULTIPLE RECORD SET
61	IDENTIFY DATA VALUES SATISFYING SPECIFIED CRITERIA IN MULTIPLE RECORD SETS

Computer Applications

With this introduction to descriptive conventions, the first computer program can be used (Program #24—Summary Table Analysis) to calculate the probability associated with that table. This program mimics operation of a sophisticated desk calculator. The entire process is as follows:

1. Dial the General Electric Information Network, using the local telephone number provided.

2. In response to U# = (shorthand for "Your user number is?"), give the number assigned. The user number represents the following:

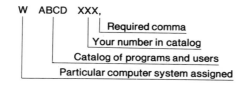

The systems are changed periodically to preserve quality of service by reorganizing the number of users on a system.

The catalog represents those users with the potential to share programs and data files. This is controlled by the catalog administrator.

The last three digits represent a particular user number with all of the rights of privacy and protection inherent in a secure system.

3. The comma following the user number is required to separate that entry from the *password.*

The password represents a special one to eight character secret word. This acts as a key to allow access to your number and is the next question asked by the computer.

4. The next entry is in response to the question

ID:

This is shorthand for *project identification.* This information is used to separate different activities within the user number.

5. The computer then executes a program which checks your status in the catalog and provides you with limited or full use of the computer, depending upon that status.

6. Full system access is identified by the message

    SYSTEM AVAILABLE

7. Issue the command

    RUN MIDAS

8. Answer the following questions as they appear (answers are underlined):

    NUMBER OF PROGRAM—? 24
    OPTION—? 3
    ROW TOTAL 1—? 10 {YOUNG}
    ROW TOTAL 2—? 10 {NOT YOUNG}
    COLUMN TOTAL 1—? 10 {MALE}
    COLUMN TOTAL 2—? 10 {FEMALE}
    FREQUENCY COLUMN 1, ROW 1—? 4 {MALE AND YOUNG}
    TABLE HEADING—? EXAMPLE
    (The table and the probability will be printed here.)
    ADDITIONAL TABLES—? 0
    NUMBER OF PROGRAM—? −1

9. BYE (Shorthand for computer disconnect instruction)

Two points need emphasis. The first involves the use of short instructions called *system commands.* Two of these were shown in the above example. At item 7, the system command RUN was used. This command, when issued in the format shown, does the following:

1. retrieves a copy of the computer program MIDAS
2. assigns control of the computer to that program
3. initiates computer function using the instructions in the program.

Item 8 involves specifications and performance associated with operation of Program 24 in MIDAS. The second system command used was at item 9. As noted there, the command BYE involves terminating connection with the computer. In addition, accounting information then will be shown. Three categories make up the cost of computer energy use. These are

1. Computer Resource Units (CRUs). Each unit represents an approxi-

mate "second" of computer activity. Computer time is not equivalent to time as we consider it. Computer time involves actual work rather than the usual process of deciding to work, organizing for it, performing it, and reviewing the product. CRUs do not reflect these work-related activities; the only accountable portion is actual work time.

2. Telephone Connect Time in Hours (TCH). This time is total, whether or not the computer is working.

3. Characters per Thousand Transmitted. Some pricing options charge for volume of transmission. This issue becomes less critical as the speed of transmitting information increases.

The accounting is continuous and is stored whether or not the command BYE is used. The command simply reports the charges to the user.

Item 8 illustrates program function requirements and performance. The specification of the program MIDAS provides the user with a variety of computing activities. In a direct sense, MIDAS is like a menu. Choice of a program in MIDAS involves selection by number. Number 24 includes four options, all related to calculating probability associated with the table entered.

Option 3 calculates the probability of a table with two rows and two columns. Probability values are decimals ranging between 0 and 1.

The usual hypothesis is that the entries in the cells will be equal in absolute or relative values. The row and column totals define the type of equality expected. With equal row and column totals, the tabular entries will be equal in absolute terms. Given that the equal frequency hypothesis is true, the relative frequency of each deviant table can be calculated. The program gives the probability value representing the observed table and those with more deviant frequencies. For example, Table 5 could represent an observed table. The probability value reported would then compute the relative frequency of tables 1, 2, 3, and 4 as well as that for 5.

1. 0 10   2. 1 9   3. 2 8
    10 0   9 1   8 2

4. 3 7   5. 4 6
    7 3   6 4

Note that all of these have the same conditions of row and column totals equal to 10.

As an exercise, the probability associated with the following tables should be computed. For option 3 (2 × 2 tables):

1. 0 5   2. 1 4   3. 2 3
    5 0   4 1   3 2

For option 4 (2 × 3 tables):

1. 0 0 5   **2.** 1 0 4   **3.** 2 0 3   **4.** 0 1 4

     5 5 0   4 5 1   3 5 2   5 4 1

Again, each table has the same row totals: row 1 = 5; row 2 = 10; and column totals: column 1 = 5; column 2 = 5; and column 3 = 5.

These two options are best used with tables having row and column totals of 20 or less. The reason for this is that, in computing the probability, the relative frequency of each extreme table leading to the one entered must be computed. Thus, a considerable amount of computing energy is involved even in what appears to be a simple problem.

This deception holds in a general fashion. That is, the easier it is for the human to understand the numeric display involved, the harder the computer works. Mathematical simplifications frequently increase the difficulty in human understanding but shorten the computer effort.

Statistics

Another computing approach illustrates the issue of the balance between human understanding and machine effort. The intent of the mathematics is to substitute one or two special numbers (statistics) for the original set of numbers. One number frequently used is called the mean or average.

The mean is computed by summing the observed values and dividing that total by the number of observations. Referring to our data summary, we will compute the mean age of the subjects entered in December of 1975. The ages are

ID Number	Age
1	30
2	25
3	40
4	53
5	37

The sum of these five ages is 30 + 25 + 40 + 53 + 37 = 185. The mean is 185/5 = 37. The location of the mean value in the set may be shown by a simple graph:

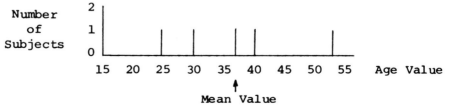

The graph shows that there is one subject respectively with age 25, 30, 37, 40, and 53. Further, the mean value is at the "center" of the observed values. The mean is used to describe sets of values because, in an arithmetic sense, it represents the central value of the set.

A second number describes the width of the set. One such descriptor is the range: Range = Largest Value *minus* Smallest Value and, in this example, is $53 - 25 = 28$. Taking the mean and range together, a description of the set would be

The central value is 37 with range 28
(smallest = 25, largest = 53).

The numbers in parenthesis represent the minimum and the maximum and assist in clarifying the appearance of the actual set of values. Four numbers rather than two were actually used.

Another way of describing width involves a modified average distance of each observed value from the mean. That is, measure the distance of each value from the mean. Average these distances. These calculations are

ID	Age	Mean	Distance
1	30	37	$(-7)^2 = 49$
2	25	37	$(-12)^2 = 144$
3	40	37	$(3)^2 = 9$
4	53	37	$(16)^2 = 256$
5	37	37	$(0)^2 = 0$
			Total = 458

Modified Average = $458/4 = 114.5$ (Divide by number of observations minus 1)

Compute square root to return to original scale:

Square Root (Modified Average) = 10.7

The distances shown are squared values of the actual differences between the value and the mean.

The Modified Average distance is called the *variance.* The square root of the variance is the *standard deviation.* When this is used with the mean, the following description of the orginal set may be given:

The central value = 37 ± 10.7.

Thus, values up to one standard deviation from the mean include those between 26.3 and 47.7. Values up to two standard deviations from the mean include those between 15.6 and 58.4. Comparing these statements with the actual set of five values shows that such summary statements are not perfect but may be adequate. The summary improves in accuracy and in usefulness as the number of values included in the set increases.

A third term similar to the standard deviation is used to describe width of mean values computed from different samples of numbers. This term is called the *standard error* and is computed by dividing the standard deviation by the square root of the number of observations used in computing the mean. For this example, the standard error is $10.7 / \sqrt{5} = 10.7/2.25 = 4.7$.

A principal use of these summary numbers is in deciding differences between samples. This is illustrated by the following example:

Compute the mean age for subjects entering the study in January 1976. The values are

ID	Age
6	44
7	16
8	69

Mean $= 44 + 16 + 69 = 129/3 = 43$.

How far away is 43 from 37 using the standard error for the December group as the ruler for measuring difference?

To answer this, take the difference and represent it in terms of standard error units. That is

$$\text{Standard Error Units} = \frac{43 - 37}{4.7} = \frac{6}{4.7} = 1.3.$$

Thus, 43 is 1.3 standard errors above 37.

Rules have been developed to assist in deciding how much difference should be seen before two samples are declared to be different. These rules are based on various ways of measuring distance. For each method, the probability calculated is associated with the question: How often would a difference as large as that one observed occur when the new sample mean is a member of the set represented by the mean and standard error used in judging difference?

Student T Test
One such method is called the Student t test. A program to compute the t statistic and the associated probability is shown (Program #30—Quick Test of Group Means). This program also mimics a desk calculator.

The complete set of system and program instructions are

1. Dial the General Electric Information Network, using the local telephone number.

2. Give: User Number
   Password
   Project Identification

3. Run MIDAS   (Answers are underlined.)

   NUMBER OF PROGRAM? 30
   NUMBER OF GROUPS? 2

   For first group:

   NAME OF GROUP? 12/75
   NUMBER OF VALUES? 5
   VALUE 1? 30
   VALUE 2? 25
   VALUE 3? 40
   VALUE 4? 53
   VALUE 5? 37

   (The mean and standard deviation for the group are displayed after the data are entered.)

   For second group:

   NAME OF GROUP? 1/76
   NUMBER OF VALUES? 3
   VALUE 1? 44
   VALUE 2? 16
   VALUE 3? 69

   (Again, the mean and standard deviation for the group are displayed.)

   COMPARE ALL GROUPS? 1 (Yes)

   (The difference in means, the t statistic, and the probability of the difference are displayed for each pair of groups compared.)

   CONTINUE WITH NEW SAMPLES? 0 (No)
   NUMBER OF PROGRAM? −1

4. Give system command BYE

The display from the program gives the means, standard deviations, t statistic, and probability value for comparing the two groups.

As an exercise, the age values for each month should be entered as a distinct group and all groups compared.

Computerized Data Management and Analysis

In an active study, manual procedures such as those already shown soon become inadequate. In the following, we will show additional computer techniques to handle new data as acquired. We will present this first by a simple translation, establishing the data summary document as a computer-readable entity. To do this requires the following system commands: NEW, SAVE, OLD, REPLACE.

The command NEW establishes a storage space (file) for information to be entered. This storage is assigned a name of your choosing. The command is used to create files which are human *and* computer readable. These files are useful in that they contain the information in a familiar form. A large number of system commands can be used to manage these files. Accordingly, without learning to program, many required data management functions are accomplished using the system commands. With the addition of the MIDAS programs, we can perform analyses, thus meeting expectations while gaining experience in computer support methods.

Following the NEW command and computer responses, type the lines of the data summary document with one additional entry at the beginning of each line. That entry is a line number. This number is used to identify storage location within the file. Line numbers can be from 1 to 5 digits in length. A common convention is to start numbering with 1000 and to increment by 5s or 10s for each subsequent line. This allows for inserting additional data records without reorganizing the file.

The data summary document, as a computer file, would be as follows:

Line Number	ID	Sex	Age	Date Entered
1000	1	1	30	751201
1010	2	1	25	751203
1020	3	1	40	751215
.	.	.	.	.
.	.	.	.	.
etc.	etc.	etc.	etc.	etc.

(Note that each new line begins with a line number and each item of data is preceded by a space.) The column headings shown are not entered into the file. Only data records are considered in our discussion.

Once all of the entries have been made, give the command SAVE. This instructs the computer to duplicate the file and put a copy into permanent storage. Only files in permanent storage are protected against loss. The command OLD retrieves from permanent storage a copy of the named file and places it in a work area called the *current file*. The command REPLACE must be used to transfer data from a current file to a previously established and permanently stored data file.

When a computer file of the data summary document has been prepared, the accuracy of data entry should be considered. For short files, verify each item by comparing it with the original paper record.

For longer files, a program in MIDAS will be of value in identifying errors. This program (#6—Verify) compares two independently prepared versions of the same data stored in separate computer files. Each discrepancy is identified.

Errors are corrected simply by retyping the indicated line. The REPLACE command transfers the corrected copy of the file to permanent storage.

Two system commands for finding and correcting data errors are: LOCATE and CHANGE.

The LOCATE command looks for and displays those records containing the pattern or string of characters specified. For example, using the following command would identify the first five records:

```
LOC   /7512/ *
                 | Display all lines with the pattern
              | Pattern to find
       | Locate command
```

The command provides considerable flexibility in search potential. Care must be exercised to describe the pattern in a unique way.

A second command, CHANGE, works in a similar fashion to LOCATE. In addition to the search, the CHANGE command also changes the pattern, once found. Suppose that the date for record 10 was to be changed from 760220 to 760222. The CHANGE command would be

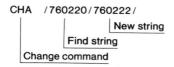

```
CHA   /760220/760222/
                   | New string
             | Find string
       | Change command
```

Written this way, the command will change only the first 760220 encountered in the file. No change is permanent until the REPLACE command is issued.

Once the data file is computerized, there are a number of programs which are helpful in analysis without being difficult to learn or use.

Analysis of a Single Variate

Program #1—Identify Data File—establishes the basic bookkeeping for the data file. Questions to be answered are

NAME OF DATA FILE?
NUMBER OF VARIATES?
NUMBER OF SUBJECTS?

Program #17—Prepare for Single Variate Distribution—is used to organize the data for display as tables and charts. The program uses either the human readable (ASCII) file or the more advanced binary file. The files constructed by Program #17 agree with the requirements of Program #18—Single Variate Distribution. This latter program provides the following displays: frequency tables, histograms, and bar graphs.

Each of these display formats is useful in describing a single variate. The frequency table answers the question: "How many?" The histogram and bar graph answer this same question, but in graphic form.

The following example illustrates the use of these two programs. The ASCII data file is as shown:

ID Number	Sex	Age
1	1	40
2	1	55
3	2	32
4	1	73
5	2	80
6	2	36
7	1	22
8	2	64
9	2	18
10	1	52
11	1	22

and consists of one record (line) for each subject. The records are read by Program #17 and the value of the age variate abstracted. These ages are stored in the second file shown:

```
     (Line number)
    ↙     ↙(Code for decimal numbers)
100    1
110    40.00   55.00    32.00   73.00   80.00      (Ages of subjects
120    36.00   22.00    64.00   18.00   52.00  ←    organized five
130    22.00   3.E+33                              values per line)
                  ↖(Code to indicate end of data)
```

This file is constructed according to the requirements of Program #18. As seen, the first line contains a line number and a code denoting that the data are decimal numbers. Lines 110 and 120 contain the age values now arranged five numbers per line. Line 130 contains the last age value and a code indicating the end of the data set.

The frequency table display from Program #18 is shown next:

SAMPLE STATISTICS FOR AGE

NO. OF OBSERVATIONS   11

AVERAGE:	44.90909
STANDARD DEVIATION:	21.40306
SMALLEST OBSERVATION:	18.00000
LARGEST OBSERVATION:	80.00000

FREQUENCY TABLE FOR AGE

CELL LOWER ENDPT	FREQ	PCT.	CUM. FREQ	CUM. PCT.
BELOW 0.				
0.	1	9.09	1	9.09
20.00	4	36.36	5	45.45
40.00	3	27.27	8	72.73
60.00	2	18.18	10	90.91
80.00	1	9.09	11	100.00

Age intervals are shown in terms of the lower value for each interval. Thus, the CELL LOWER ENDPT column means:

From	but not equal	To
0		20
20		40
40		60
60		80
80		Infinity

The first value shown, BELOW 0, is given to indicate the number of values below the range considered.

Comparing the frequency table with the data file:

The Interval Lower Endpoint			Number	Values
0	to	20	1	18 (ID 9)
20		40	4	32,36,22,22
etc.				(IDs 3,6,7,11)

the frequency table program reports:

FREQ : the number of values in the interval

PCT   : the percent of the total in the interval

CUM FREQ : the total number of values from all intervals less than and equal to the current one

CUM PCT : the percent of the total from all intervals less than and equal to the current one.

These programs, #17 and #18, provide considerable computer support using the ASCII data file. This data management approach works best when the data record is relatively small (one or two lines) and there is only one record per subject.

Removing Permanent Files
The PURGE command enables you to remove from permanent storage those files which are no longer needed.

Program #81 in MIDAS also may be used to purge files.

Summary
Basic ingredients to perform data management and analysis include

1.   Data Management Concepts
    a.   Variate List
    b.   Data Recording Document
    c.   Data Summary Document
       1)   Paper Version
       2)   ASCII File Version
    d.   System Commands
       1)   NEW (FILE NAME)
       2)   SAVE—New File
       3)   OLD (FILE NAME)
       4)   REPLACE—Old File
       5)   PURGE (FILE NAME)
       6)   RUN
       7)   LOCATE
       8)   CHANGE
    e.   Programs
       1)   VERIFY (Program #6)
       2)   PURGE (Program #81)
2.   Analytical Concepts
    a.   Immediate—No Stored Data

1) SUMMARY TABLE ANALYSES (Program #24, options 3 and 4)
2) QUICK TEST OF GROUP MEANS (Program #30)

b. Data File Prepared—ASCII Type
1) IDENTIFY DATA FILE (Program #1)
2) PREPARE FOR SINGLE VARIATE DISTRIBUTION (Program #17)
3) SINGLE VARIATE DISTRIBUTION (Program #18)
4) STOP MIDAS (Program #−1)

Section 2

Management Procedures with Direct Access Binary Files

The human readable (ASCII) file as the basis for computer-supported data management and analysis offers considerable improvement in study conduct potential in comparison to paper files and manual methods. Indeed, the relatively small study (100 subjects or less) with data records of one to two lines per subject could be successfully managed using the procedures outlined in Section 1. The analytical approaches with the ASCII file are limited in MIDAS primarily because it is expensive to use this inefficient storage method.

The ability to manage an ASCII file data base successfully decreases as the individual data record increases in size; as the number of subjects exceeds small study limits; and as the study increases in operational complexity. A frequent example of this last point is the situation where

1. The number of different record types (independently obtained sets of variates) increases. Examples of different record types are
    a. Characteristics measured at entry into the study (a prestudy record);
    b. Characteristics measured at some critical time in the study (an event record).

2. The completion and reporting of these different record types do not conform to an ordered sequence. For example, prestudy records are not reported in the sequence reflecting the consecutive entry of subjects into the study, even though the data are captured in the appropriate sequence. This "breakdown" in reporting, from the investigators to the data management group, is a phenomenon which can occur frequently. Thus, the data management process must be able to accommodate to the sequence of reported prestudy records such as:

5, 2, 7, 1, 6, 3, 9, 4, . . . , as well as the sequence: 1, 2, 3, 4, 5, 6, 7, 8, 9, ... The numbers in the sequences represent IDs assigned to subjects as they enter the study.

An additional complication is the reporting of other record types in various non-ordered arrangements. As the number of different records increases, insertion of each into its ASCII data file involves more time and effort. Opportunities to make "filing errors" also increase.

Direct Access Binary Files and Data Management

At this point, a simple approach involving essentially the same data management concepts as in Section 1 is presented. The change is in the type of file used to store the basic data. Data management difficulties with the ASCII file type can be summarized as those associated with the filing process. The identification of the proper location for inserting or retrieving a record becomes more difficult to accomplish. To alleviate this, the basic data file should be *direct access binary* rather than ASCII.

As the name implies, the direct access binary file is constructed to enable the selection of a record position to store or retrieve records. Adopting the convention that the ID number (the study sequence number) assigned to the subject upon entry is equivalent to the record position in the direct access file allows easy storage and retrieval. For example, the sequence of prestudy records described earlier was 5, 2, 7, 1, 6, 3, 9, 4, ... These data records could be computerized by constructing an ASCII file as follows:

**Format of ASCII File Used to Enter Data
Records into Direct Access Binary File**

Line Number	ID Number	Sex	Age	Date Entered Study
1000	5	2	37	751231
1005	2	1	25	751203
1010	7	1	16	760122
1015	1	1	30	751201
1020	6	2	44	760109
1025	3	1	40	751215
1030	9	1	72	760212
1035	4	1	53	751226

*(These data records are the same as those given
in Section 1.)*

In this ASCII file, the first thing to notice is that the line numbers are increased to enter the records as reported rather than to reflect study entry as in Section 1.

A further distinction in the use of ASCII files is also illustrated. This file was *not* constructed as the basic data management vehicle but rather as a temporary bridge connecting the paper report with the basic direct access binary file. When a file serves in this temporary capacity, it is designated as a "holding file." Once the data records have been transferred to the permanent file structure, holding files are purged.

The "loading" operations performed by the MIDAS programs involve:

1. reading the holding file, one record at a time
2. identifying the ID number value
3. selecting the record position in the direct access file corresponding to the ID number value
4. storing the data record in that position of the file.

These steps imply that the direct access file must contain a record position for each possible ID number. A further condition in this file design is that each record be of the same fixed length. Thus, at any given point in time in the study, there will be empty records (all zero values except for the ID number). These records represent those subjects for whom the data have not been reported. To illustrate this, consider what the direct access file would look like after loading of the holding file.

Format of Direct Access Binary Basic Data File

Position ID Number	Sex	Age	Date Entered Study
1	1	30	751201
2	1	25	751203
3	1	40	751215
4	1	53	751226
5	2	37	751231
6	2	44	760109
7	1	16	760122
8	0	0	0
9	1	72	760212

Note that the record at position 8 is zero, except for the ID number.

Program #3 Data Management Options

To manage records in this system, we will construct a direct access file for each record type. In this way, we will be able to

1. store records presented in any order within record type
2. identify "missing" (zero value) records within record type
3. perform analyses with each file separately
4. merge the data records for each subject in order to prepare analyses across record types.

Data management procedures for the direct access file are integrated into one program (Program #3). To illustrate the use of this program, we will deal with each function separately.

Example 1 **Create Direct Access File and Load First Records**

NUMBER OF PROGRAM? 1   *(Identify file)*
NAME OF DATA FILE? NAME   *(Name of ASCII holding file)*
NUMBER OF VARIATES? 4   *(In prestudy file)*
NUMBER OF SUBJECTS? 8   *(Number of records in holding file)*

NUMBER OF PROGRAM? 3   *(Data management)*
DATA MANAGEMENT OPTION? 1   *(Load data from ASCII file)*
NUMBER OF LINES PER RECORD? 1   *(1 line per subject in ASCII file)*
NAME OF DIRECT ACCESS FILE? DATA   *(Any name)*
CREATE OR LENGTHEN FILE? 1   *(Option to create new file)*
MAXIMUM ID NUMBER? 9   *(Established size of file initially)*

Example 2 **With the Direct Access File Created, Additional Records Are Entered from a New Holding File As Follows:**

NUMBER OF PROGRAM? 1
NAME OF DATA FILE? NAME
NUMBER OF VARIATES? 4   *(Identify data file)*
NUMBER OF SUBJECTS? 1

NUMBER OF PROGRAM? 3
DATA MANAGEMENT OPTION? 1
NUMBER OF LINES PER RECORD? 1
NAME OF DIRECT ACCESS FILE? DATA
CREATE OR LENGTHEN FILE? 3   *(Use file without lengthening)*
MAXIMUM ID NUMBER? 9

Example 3 **When the File Is to Be Increased in Length:**

NUMBER OF PROGRAM? 1
NAME OF DATA FILE? NAME
NUMBER OF VARIATES? 4   *(Identify data file)*
NUMBER OF SUBJECTS? 11

NUMBER OF PROGRAM? 3
DATA MANAGEMENT OPTION? 1

NUMBER OF LINES?   1

NAME OF DIRECT ACCESS FILE?   DATA

CREATE OR LENGTHEN FILE?   2   *(Option to increase length)*

MAXIMUM ID NUMBER?   20   *(File size increased to hold 20 records)*

Example 4 To List Records Stored in File:

NUMBER OF PROGRAM?   1 ⎤

NAME OF DATA FILE?   DATA ⎥

NUMBER OF VARIATES?   4   *(Identify data file)*

NUMBER OF SUBJECTS?   20 ⎦

NUMBER OF PROGRAM?   16   *(Define subgroups)*

NAME OF COVARIATE DEFINITION FILE?   COVLOOK   *(Any name)*

NUMBER OF NEW PROBLEMS?   2

PROBLEM NUMBER?   1   *(Find zero records)*

NUMBER OF COVARIATES?   1

VARIATE NUMBER?   4   *(Use date variate to identify zero record)*

LOWER BOUND, UPPER BOUND?   −.5, .5

PROBLEM NUMBER?   2   *(Find records for December entries)*

NUMBER OF COVARIATES?   1

VARIATE NUMBER?   4

LOWER BOUND, UPPER BOUND?   751201, 751231

NUMBER OF PROGRAM?   3

DATA MANAGEMENT OPTION?   2   *(List records)*

LIST SUBSET OF VARIATES?   *(Y= 1; N= 0)*   0

POSITION?   1   *(First record)*

 (Data record for ID 1 listed here)

POSITION?   0   *(Stop individual record listing)*

NUMBER OF PROGRAM?   3

DATA MANAGEMENT OPTION?   2

LIST SUBSET OF VARIATES?   0

POSITION?   −1   *(List all records)*

COVARIATE PROBLEM NUMBER?   1   *(Zero record subgroup)*

 (Data records for missing entries listed. ID numbers are displayed together with zero entries for other variates.)

Example 5 To Correct Records Stored in File:

NUMBER OF PROGRAM?   1 ⎤

NAME OF DATA FILE?   DATA ⎥

NUMBER OF VARIATES?   4   *(Identify data file)*

NUMBER OF SUBJECTS?   20 ⎦

NUMBER OF PROGRAM? 3

DATA MANAGEMENT OPTION? 3 *(Correct variate option)*

POSITION? 1 *(Location of record to be corrected)*

NUMBER OF CORRECTIONS? 1

VARIATE NUMBER, NEW VALUE? 3, 29 *(Change age to 29)*

POSITION? 0 *(Stop corrections)*

Example 6 To Prepare an Analytical Copy of the Data Management File:

The MIDAS analytical programs use a binary file type constructed for efficiency in dealing with *all* of the data records. This is in contrast to the *single* record emphasis in data management. This analytical file type is called the FAST file in MIDAS. The data management oriented direct access file is called the SLOW file. As will be shown in the next section, the FAST file is used with a number of data management functions involving rapid processing of the data records, as well as in analytical programs. Preparation of the analytical copy of the data is as follows:

NUMBER OF PROGRAM? 1

NAME OF DATA FILE? DATA

NUMBER OF VARIATES? 4 *(Identify file)*

NUMBER OF SUBJECTS? 20

NUMBER OF PROGRAM? 16

NAME OF COVARIATE DEFINITION FILE? COVLOOK

NUMBER OF NEW PROBLEMS? 1

PROBLEM NUMBER? 3 *(Select non-zero records using date of entry variate)*

NUMBER OF COVARIATES? 1

VARIATE NUMBER? 4

LOWER BOUND, UPPER BOUND? 751201, 760630

(Define covariate subgroup)

NUMBER OF PROGRAM? 3

DATA MANAGEMENT OPTION? 4 *(Create analytical file)*

NAME OF ANALYTICAL FILE? COMPUTE *(Any name)*

COVARIATE PROBLEM NUMBER? 3 *(Select only non-zero records for analysis)*

Summary

Program #3 performs the essential data management functions associated with an individual record. New records are added from an ASCII holding file. Data records may be corrected either by reentering the data using a record in the ASCII file or by using the correct value option in Program #3. Data records may be listed using the list option. Individual records, subsets satisfying covariate rules, or all records can be displayed. The final option allows for the construction of a special copy of the data file. This copy, the fast or analytical file, is used in analyses and in file management procedures requiring rapid processing of all of the data records in a file.

Data management using the slow file introduced in this section offers the advantage of ease in storing and retrieving individual records. The direct access capability provides the desired ordering of the records irrespective of the sequence entered. The ordering of data records provides the capability of identifying and displaying study progress in a straightforward fashion. As such, this management approach represents use and cost improvements over ASCII file based procedures.

The ASCII file is now used in an efficient fashion as a temporary reservoir for records during the communication process. Once the data are confirmed, the conversion of the ASCII to binary simplifies all further computing functions.

Section 3

The Analytical Data File

The purpose of this section is to illustrate the use of the analytical data file. This file type is a special form of the direct access binary file. It is constructed by appropriate MIDAS programs. The design used facilitates storage and retrieval of *sections* of the file. Each section contains many complete data records.

The primary reason for using the analytical data file is economy. The slowest step in computing is the communication between the computer and peripheral equipment. These communications are reduced in number by dealing with multiple records. The analytical file construction allows for faster performance than does the ASCII file (Section 1) or the direct access binary file (Section 2). This file type is called FAST in the MIDAS programs.

The file design also offers convenience. Manual summaries of the data (as in Section 1) can be performed by the computer, once mechanisms for reducing costs are available. A third benefit is accuracy because, once data files are prepared and verified, the probability of machine error is considerably smaller than for human error.

Creating the Fast File

The analytical file should always represent a *copy* of the basic data file. The fast file may be prepared either from an ASCII file (Program #2) or from a direct access binary file (Program #3). The instructions for copying the direct access file were shown in Section 2. The instructions for copying an ASCII file are

NUMBER OF PROGRAM? <u>1</u>		
NAME OF DATA FILE? <u>NAME</u>	*(Identify ASCII file)*	
NUMBER OF VARIATES? <u>4</u>		
NUMBER OF SUBJECTS? <u>10</u>		

NUMBER OF PROGRAM? <u>2</u> *(Copy ASCII to FAST)*
NUMBER OF LINES PER RECORD? <u>1</u> *(in ASCII file)*
NAME OF FAST BINARY FILE? <u>FAST</u> *(any name)*

Records written into the FAST file will be in exactly the same order as in the ASCII file. The restrictions in constructing the fast copy are

1. numerical data only
2. equal number of variates per record.

The conversion from ASCII to binary file formats is illustrated as follows:

**Format of ASCII File Used to Enter Data
Records into Direct Access Binary File**

Line Number	ID Number	Sex	Age	Date Entered Study
1000	5	2	37	751231
1005	2	1	25	751203
1010	7	1	16	760122
1015	1	1	30	751201
1020	6	2	44	760109
1025	3	1	40	751215
1030	9	1	72	760212
1035	4	1	53	751226

↓

Format of Fast Analytical File

ID Number	Sex	Age	Date Entered Study
5	2	37	751231
2	1	25	751203
7	1	16	760122
1	1	30	751201
6	2	44	760109
3	1	40	751215
9	1	72	760212
4	1	53	751226

Data Display Analyses

The programs to be described were first introduced in Section 1 with the ASCII file. Display programs (Programs #17 and #18) also may be used with the fast file. Program #17 is chosen to prepare the data for subsequent analysis. The instructions associated with the fast file would be

NUMBER OF PROGRAM? <u>17</u> *(Prepare for data display)*
FILE TYPE? <u>1</u> *(Use fast file)*

```
USE ZERO VALUES?  (Y= 1;N= 0)  0  (Ignore "zero" values)
NUMBER OF INPUT FILES?  2  (See discussion below)
VARIATE NUMBER?  2 {SEX}  (Variate chosen)
INPUT FILE NAME?  SEX  (Any name)
SAVE OUTPUT FROM DISPLAY PROGRAMS IN A FILE?  (Y= 1;N= 0)  0
VARIATE NUMBER?  3 {AGE}  (Variate chosen)
INPUT FILE NAME?  AGE  (Any name)
```

Program #17 is used to prepare data files (ASCII in type) consisting of a single variate organized according to the requirements of Program #18. This is done by selecting the variate value from each record in the data file and by stringing these values out in a line, five per line, as follows:

```
(Line number)
   ╱    (Code for decimal numbers)
100   1
110   40.00   55.00   32.00   73.00   80.00 ⎤  (Ages of subjects organized
120   36.00   22.00   64.00   18.00   52.00 ⎥ ← five values per line)
130   22.00   3.E+33                         ⎦
               ╲ (Code to indicate end of data)
```

This new file is used to supply the data to Program #18.

In general, *input* is information supplied to a program; *output* is information provided by a program. Since the purpose of Program #17 is to prepare files for Program #18, it is appropriate to use the term *input* to describe the type of file developed by Program #17.

Program #18 can be instructed to write the analytical displays into *output* files. If desired, these output files will be created in Program #17 as empty space ready to receive the analytical results.

Means and Student T Tests

Program #30 (Quick Test for Means) was introduced in Section 1 to enable the calculation of means, standard deviations, Student t tests, and associated probabilities for the comparison of groups. When the number of variates per record and the number of records exceed desk calculator dimensions, the MIDAS Programs #1, #26, #28, and #29 offer an efficient alternative approach.

Suppose the problem involves comparing ages of subjects entered before 760301 (one subgroup) with those for subjects entered after that date. The instructions would be as follows:

```
NUMBER OF PROGRAM?  1   ⎤
NAME OF DATA FILE?  FAST ⎥
NUMBER OF VARIATES?  4   ⎥ (Identify fast copy of data)
NUMBER OF SUBJECTS?  20  ⎦
```

NUMBER OF PROGRAM? 16
NAME OF COVARIATE DEFINITION FILE? <u>ANY</u>   *(Any name)*
NUMBER OF NEW PROBLEMS? <u>2</u>
PROBLEM NUMBER? <u>1</u>   *(Records < 760301 for entry date)*
NUMBER OF COVARIATES? <u>1</u>
VARIATE NUMBER? <u>4</u>
LOWER BOUND, UPPER BOUND? <u>751130, 760229</u>
PROBLEM NUMBER? <u>2</u>   *(Records ≥ 760301)*
NUMBER OF COVARIATES? <u>1</u>
VARIATE NUMBER? <u>4</u>
LOWER BOUND, UPPER BOUND? <u>760301, 770101</u>

NUMBER OF PROGRAM? <u>26</u>   *(Calculate MEANS for 1st subgroup)*
USE ZERO VALUES? *(Y= 1;N= 0)* <u>0</u>   *(No zero values used)*
COVARIATE PROBLEM NUMBER? <u>1</u>   *(Select only records < 760301)*
PRINT MEANS? *(Y= 1;N= 0)* <u>1</u>
   (Means, Standard Deviations, and Sample Sizes printed here)

NUMBER OF PROGRAM? <u>28</u>   *(Prepare for t test)*
OPTION? <u>3</u>   *(Select subset of variates)*
NUMBER OF VARIATES IN SUBSET? <u>1</u>
VARIATE 1? <u>3</u>   *(Age)*
NUMBER OF SAMPLE? <u>1</u>   *(First subgroup processed)*
ADDITIONAL SAMPLES? *(Y= 1;N= 0)* <u>1</u>

NUMBER OF PROGRAM? <u>26</u>   *(Calculate MEANS for 2nd subgroup)*
USE ZERO VALUES? *(Y= 1;N= 0)* <u>0</u>
COVARIATE PROBLEM NUMBER? <u>2</u>   *(Select only records ≥ 760301)*
PRINT MEANS? *(Y= 1;N= 0)* <u>1</u>
   (Second group calculations printed here)

NUMBER OF PROGRAM? <u>28</u>   *(Prepare for t test)*
OPTION? <u>3</u>   *(Select subset of variates)*
NUMBER OF VARIATES IN SUBSET? <u>1</u>
VARIATE 1? <u>3</u>   *(Age)*
NUMBER OF SAMPLE? <u>2</u>   *(Second subgroup processed)*
ADDITIONAL SAMPLES? *(Y= 1;N= 0)* <u>0</u>

NUMBER OF PROGRAM? <u>29</u>   *(Compute Student t tests)*
USE FILE - INPUT? *(Y= 1;N= 0)* <u>1</u>   *(File prepared by Program #28)*
OPTION? <u>1</u>   *(Compare group means)*
NUMBER OF GROUPS COMPARED? <u>2</u>
COMPARE ALL GROUPS? *(Y= 1;N= 0)* <u>1</u>
   (Results printed here)

As seen, the covariate option is used in selecting the records for each group. The mean, standard deviation, and number of observations (sample size) are calculated for each variate—ID, sex, age, and date entered— even though we are only interested in age. It is more effective to compute the statistics on all variates in the record. The reasons for this are

1. The fast file can be processed quickly with the complete variate list relative to selection of specific variates for storage in a separate file.
2. Variates of interest can be selected from a statistical summary file prepared by the MEANS program. The file is called MEANS and is ASCII in type. The format is

MEAN VALUE, STANDARD DEVIATION, SAMPLE SIZE

for each variate in the record. No line numbers are used.

Note that Program #28 (Prepare for t test) actually reads the MEANS file and selects the third variate—mean age, standard deviation of age, and sample size of age—for storage in a second file called INPUT. This file will contain, for each subgroup chosen, the statistics associated with the variates to be compared in the Student t Test program (#29). The file INPUT has the following format:

LINE NUMBER, MEAN, STANDARD DEVIATION, SAMPLE SIZE

for each variate in Group 1. Statistics for Group 2 are entered after Group 1, and so on.

Two issues need emphasis. The first is associated with the computation of statistics for a group. These statistics—mean, standard deviation, and sample size for each variate—are stored in the MEANS file. This file will be purged each time Program #26 is requested and when MIDAS is stopped (Program # − 1). If the statistics should be saved, use Program #80 (Convert Files for Long-Term Storage) to create a binary copy of MEANS.

The second issue is that, once the MEANS file has been prepared for a group and saved under a user-defined name (Program #80), it can be used in programs requiring the statistics by instructing Program #80 to reverse the copy procedure.

Files such as MEANS, and others to be described later, represent considerable savings in computing in that, once performed for a group, there is no need to recompute the statistics again. This is in contrast to other programming systems which frequently involve recomputing these statistics as each analytical program is chosen. This is wasteful effort and more expensive. To take advantage of the MIDAS savings, statistical summary files such as MEANS must be saved using a name chosen by the user.

Tabular Analyses: The Chi-Square Statistic

In Section 1, relationships between two variates were explored using Program #24 and the option for exact tests of contingency tables. An alternative approach with larger samples uses the chi-square statistic to test for relationships. This statistic and its associated probability are provided by two programs in MIDAS—#22, the 2 × 2 table; and #23, the 10 × 10 (maximum size) table.

The discussion in Section 1 of subgroups, boundary values, etc., applies to these programs as well. The difference is that Programs #22 and #23 build the tables by reading the fast file. No manual summarization is required.

Interpreting the chi-square and probability requires explanation. The chi-square statistic is computed using the concept of expected frequencies as well as the observed frequencies in each cell of the table. Using an example similar to that in Section 1 for the two by two table, the data might be as follows:

		Column 1	2	Total
Row	1	20	5	25
	2	5	20	25
	Total	25	25	50

The numbers shown are the observed frequencies. The expected frequencies, if the two variates were totally unrelated, would be

		Column 1	2	Total
Row	1	12.5	12.5	25
	2	12.5	12.5	25
	Total	25.0	25.0	50

Note that no relationship means equal frequency in each cell for this example. The chi-square statistic involves assessment of the *distance* between the observed and expected for each cell, relative to the expected frequency as the measure of distance. That is

$$\text{Chi-square} = \frac{(20 - 12.5)^2}{12.5} \quad \frac{\textit{Distance 1st cell}}{\textit{Expected frequency 1st cell}}$$

$$+ \frac{(5 - 12.5)^2}{12.5} \quad \frac{\textit{Distance 2nd cell}}{\textit{Expected frequency 2nd cell}}$$

$$+ \frac{(5 - 12.5)^2}{12.5} \quad \textit{etc.}$$

$$+ \frac{(20 - 12.5)^2}{12.5} \quad \textit{etc.}$$

Since each cell or subgroup is independent, the relative distances can be summed to determine the total chi-square value. The probability associated with the chi-square statistic is computed assuming that the observed table is a sample from the expected frequency table. If the observed table deviates from the expected, the probability will be small (close to zero). The smaller the probability value, the more the observed deviates from expectation. This phenomenon is considered significant if the probability value is less than 0.05. A table with small probability should always be visually checked to verify the relationship shown by the observed data. If a relationship is not obvious, check the instructions to confirm their accuracy. Mistakes in data files and / or in instructions could also give rise to significant results.

Summary

The purpose of this section was to introduce the fast file for those computations shown in Section 1. The distinction between the use of the ASCII file and the fast file in Program #17 is one of cost. The fast file is constructed to allow rapid processing of the records and is thus cheaper.

This economy in processing represents a continuing reason for using the fast file through the analytical component of the MIDAS set of programs. Other cost savings are associated with the use of files such as MEANS, a statistical summary file.

The other advantage to the fast file is convenience. That is, summaries of the data—performed manually in Section 1—can be performed by the computer, once mechanisms for reducing costs have been developed. A note of caution is appropriate in that, as more effort is shifted to the computer, the apparent costs will increase. Real costs can be identified only when manual procedures are assigned appropriate monetary values.

The MIDAS programs have been constructed to work with those file types offering economy in performance. The system also is constructed to offer flexibility in choice, where practical. When the programs insist on using the fast file type, it is because substantial savings are possible. The major purpose of the modular approach is to offer computing and data management capability in the most competitive and efficient fashion available. One of the adjustments required by the data manager is attention to the file design as it relates to the problems to be solved. A valuable tool is the fast file construction, as it allows for more rapid processing of large files than other designs. The MIDAS programs will deviate from this file type only when some other requirement becomes more pressing.

Section 4

Changing Data Values

The need to change data values will arise after the data preparation and verification process. Changing values may actually involve

1. correction of specific values of variates in certain data records
2. changing specific values of variates in all records
3. changing all values of variates in all records.

The purpose of this section is to illustrate those programs involved in providing the changes.

Program #7 Correction of Specific Data
This program provides the mechanism for changing variate values in the fast file. While it is convenient to make corrections in this file to continue the analysis, one must be careful. The fast file should be a *copy* of the basic data file (in ASCII or slow binary form). Correction should then also be made in the basic data record.

Occasionally, a user will decide to make the fast file his basic data repository. It is possible and most convenient to do this when all data for a study have been computerized. Updating of fast files for ongoing studies can be done using the programs discussed in the next section. However, until the user feels confident in his knowledge of file management mechanisms, the correction program (X7) and the others to be presented in this section should be considered as part of the *analytical* capabilities.

Program #7 requires knowledge of the location of each record to be changed. Note that, in Section 2, the position of a record in the slow file conformed to the ID number assigned to the subject upon entry. This agreement between ID number and file position means that locations of records were always known. The sequence of record storage in the fast file conforms to the order of the ASCII or slow binary used in its creation. This order may or may not conform to an ID number sequence.

Program #7 is designed to provide a listing of record locations and ID numbers. This listing may include all or a specific subset of subjects' records as defined by a covariate problem stored in the covariate definition file. The listing will be displayed at the terminal or in an ASCII file named by the user. If the file option is chosen, the program transfers control back to the menu (MIDAS), as corrections are not possible until the ASCII file is listed. Display of positions at the terminal allows the program to continue.

Once positions are known, the program requires the same information as shown in Section 2, as follows:

POSITION? <u>2</u>   *(Record location)*
NUMBER OF CORRECTIONS? <u>1</u>
VARIATE NUMBER, NEW VALUE? <u>3, 29</u>   *(Change age from original value to 29)*

POSITION? <u>0</u> *(No further corrections)*

The corrected data are stored in the same analytical file.

Program #12 Calendar Date Conversion

Dates may be stored in the data record in one of two formats:

1.   As three two-digit variates arranged as month, day, year.

     This format should be used for all dates prior to March 1, 1900, and when any segment of the total date is missing.

     If both month and year are recorded as zero, the date conversion will be made zero, as it is assumed that the date is missing. If the year value is greater than the current year, the date is assumed to be from the previous century. Date conversion will take place as long as the year is not zero. The month must be greater than zero if the year is zero.

2.   As one variate arranged YYMMDD. This date presentation allows for only actual values: 751231 is correct; 760100 is incorrect.

     In addition, this format may be used only for dates after March 1, 1900.

The first step in date conversion in both date formats is to change to serial days. The two formats give scales which are *different* and *cannot be used together.* Each format may be used to compute time changes between dates. Time changes computed between dates, using different formats, will be *wrong.*

An example using both date conversion and time change follows.

Suppose the data records were

ID Number	Sex	Age	Date Entered	Date of Event
1	1	40	751201	760301
2	1	50	751202	760402
3	2	45	751210	760225
.	.	.	.	.
.	.	.	.	.
etc.	etc.	etc.	etc.	etc.

Instructions for using Program #12 are

OPTION? 2   *(Convert dates and time changes)*
NUMBER OF DATES TO CONVERT? 2
DATE FORMAT? 2   *(YYMMDD format)*
VARIATE NUMBER–DATE 1? 4   *(Date entered)*
VARIATE NUMBER–DATE 2? 5   *(Date of event)*
NUMBER OF TIME CHANGES? 1
BASELINE VARIATE, OTHER TIME VARIATE? 6, 7   *(See below)*
TIME CALCULATION OPTION? 1   *(Calculate difference in days)*

Each converted date is stored as a *new* variate in the record. Accordingly, variate 4, the date entered, is changed to serial days and stored in the first available location—6. Variate 5, the date of the event, is converted to serial days and stored in the next location—7. The difference between these serial day values is computed in days and stored in the next available location—8. The increased record is stored back into the FAST file. The serial day conversions are stored as part of the record in the event that they are needed at some later place in the analysis. This is particularly helpful when a large number of dates are being converted and a relatively small number of time changes calculated.

Program #13 Recode Data Values
This program is of value in the following situations:

1. The record contains variate locations for a number of possible events.
    Each of the events is identified by a date. It is possible for a given individual to experience none, one, or more than one of these events. Further, the events can be ordered according to importance. The problem to be resolved requires searching through the ordered date variates to find the first non-zero one. This date would be transferred to the location used to record occurrence of events. Analysis of the

"events" variate would describe the time to occurrence of the first of a set of possible events experienced by each subject.

2.   The record contains variates with values to be changed.
        Here the need is to change all variate 1 values of 50 to 1, all variate 1 values of 55 to 2, etc. This process is consistent with the descriptive word, recode. The mechanism is useful in changing numbers for descriptive purposes to various scaled indices.

Program #14 Transformations

The program makes it possible to alter the scales represented by the variates. Scale changes are accomplished by changing each value to

1.   The logarithm of the value.
        This transformation tends to reduce the width of a number set. The program computes *natural* logarithms.

2.   The anti-logarithm of the value.
        This transformation converts the log scale back to the original scale.

3.   The square root of the value.
        This transformation also tends to shrink the scale. For example, the numbers 4, 9, 16 would be changed to 2, 3, 4.

4.   The variate raised to a power.
        This transformation expands the scale. For the power of 2, the numbers 2, 3, 4 would be 4, 9, 16.

5.   The inverse of the value.
        This transformation involves dividing the number 1 by the variate value. A large value gives a small inverse value (say, $1/1000 = 0.001$); a small value gives a large inverse value (say, $1/0.001 = 1000$).

In addition, the program provides for simple computations of these variates:

1.   a variate plus or minus a constant
2.   a variate multiplied or divided by a constant
3.   the sum, difference, product, or quotient of two variates.

The transformation program operates on all variate values except zeros. The latter value is assumed, throughout the MIDAS system, to be a missing value. If zeros are legitimate values, they should be transformed using the "variate plus constant" option to some small number such as 0.0001; that is, the constant would be 0.0001. The analytical programs provide the option of including or excluding zero values from the analysis.

Summary

The programs described in this section involve the "change value" concept and operate on records stored in a fast file. Changing values is important for analytical capability rather than for data management.

The fast file is used to reduce costs of these variate value change procedures. Note, however, that, while working with one record is possible in Program #7 (Correct Data Values), the other programs "work" on all records satisfying specified conditions. The economic hazards associated with inexperience in computer operations shrink as these and future programs are introduced. The binary file constructed to allow for selection of many records at one time does not prevent effective file management. Indeed, for the informed person, this file type provides all that is available with either the ASCII or slow binary, and at less cost.

Section 5

Management Procedures with the Analytical File

Introduction

Additional file management programs using the analytical or fast binary file are discussed in this section. These programs are of value in preparing data records for a variety of analyses. In contrast to programs presented in Section 4, these produce a new binary file with the altered data.

In addition, a new type of binary file is introduced in this section. This new type of file satisfies a specific purpose. In many analytical exercises there is a distinct need for *scratch paper*. The new type, *sequential binary*, is used in lieu of scratch paper. The file is constructed so that records are stored and retrieved without regard to order except for the "first come, first stored" rule. This construction is useful in many situations, particularly where large numbers of records must be processed quickly for retrieval or storage.

As indicated above, a new data file is prepared as a result of the program. The new file name, number of variates, and number of records become the current information maintained in the MIDAS system. It is important to keep this switch in files in mind, particularly when considering covariate problems with further analysis. Note that covariate problems are identified by variates and specific variate values. As the data file changes, the covariate problem must agree with the current data record to function correctly.

Program #8 Append Data Files

This program prepares a new fast file incorporating records of the same length from two files. The files are appended in the order specified. This operation is useful in investigating multi-group questions after each subgroup has been analyzed. Again, the data file and dimensions are changed to those representing the new one.

Program #11 Select Records and Variates

This program prepares a new fast file containing records which satisfy one of the following options:

1. An altered list of variates for all records in the original file.

    The new list has a maximum of 100 variates. The variates may be arranged in any order. A typical use of this option is to select a smaller set of variates. Another is to extend the variate list by repeating certain variates. This is helpful in some recode or transformation applications. For example:

    a. Recode AGE to specified values

    The variate AGE could be included in this selected list twice: once to preserve the actual value for use in further analyses, the second time in recoding of the form—change 30 to 40 to 1, etc. This variate, recoded, could be used in other analyses.

    b. Calculate the ratio of height to age

    The transformation program stores the changed value in the orginal location for the variate. When two variates are used, the changed value is stored in the location of the first variate specified. If the original variate is to be retrieved along with the transformed variate, the select program should be used. In this situation, the variate HEIGHT would be specified twice. One would be used in the transformation program for calculation of height divided by age; the other would be used to preserve the original height value.

2. A subset of records containing the original list of variates (maximum of 1500 records in new file)

    This option provides the mechanism to satisfy the requirement for choosing and retaining a subgroup of records. The option is conceptually the same as that used in covariate selection. The distinction is in retention of the records. If the records are to be used in an extensive analysis, it is more efficient and cheaper to select them once and to use the file containing only those records in the analysis. Note that covariate selection uses the original file to select the records of interest. Repeated selection of a small subset from a big file could be accomplished by covariate definition. However, even with fast files, that operation is not as efficient as doing it once in the select program.

3. A combination of variate and record selection

    This option allows for the development of an altered list of variates in a subset of records. This is appropriate when extensive analyses are planned involving the variates chosen for the subset of records.

This program automatically changes the bookkeeping of the data file. The new file name, number of variates, and number of records replace the original file information.

Program #9 Merge Data Files
The merge program takes data records from two fast files, matches the ID numbers, and prepares a *new record* consisting of the two original records. The second ID number is dropped from the new record. This program is useful in adding data to an existing record. *Only those records with data from both files are included in the merged file.*

Program #10 Sort Data Records
The sort program takes data records from ASCII files (no line numbers), slow or fast binary files, and from the new sequential binary files. In this format, records are stored or retrieved in the order presented. No attempt is made to sequence records as stored, and the rule is "first come, first served." The sequential binary file type is ideal for scratch paper operations and is used in MIDAS for that purpose. Conversion from sequential to other forms will be described.

The sort program is used to rearrange data records in a requested way. The ordering is accomplished by specifying the variates to be used in arranging the records. Variates used in this fashion are called "sort keys." Rules for sorting are

1. Arrange records using first sort key.
2. If ties in value of first key, use second key to break ties, etc.

All records are retained, including ties.

Program #4 Convert Binary Files
This program provides a mechanism to change from one type of binary file to another. Each type of binary file serves a specific purpose and each is chosen to minimize cost. This program provides for the conversion from

1. fast to sequential
2. fast to slow
3. sequential to fast
4. slow to fast.

Program #5 Convert Binary File to ASCII File
This program allows any of the binary files to be converted back to the ASCII file. In preparing the ASCII record, the data values can be stored as integers or as decimal numbers. A format statement can be prepared or program format statements provided. The format statement is an instruction for arrangement of the numbers in the record.

1. An integer-oriented format statement
    Format statements begin with an open parenthesis. Spacing between numbers is controlled by the use of the letter X. Thus, 1X is one space, 2X is 2 spaces, etc. Integer numbers are denoted by the letter I. The

width of the number also must be given. In describing integer numbers, the group I3 would represent numbers from 00 to ±99, I4 for 000 to ±999, etc. Multiple numbers of the same width would be described by 2I3, which stands for two numbers each three characters wide. Variates in the ASCII file should be separated by a space. To accomplish this, use: 2 (I3,1X), which stands for two arrangements, where each consists of a three-character integer number followed by a space. When the format instruction is completed, a close parenthesis, is used. Some examples are

    a. (3(I3,1X),I4)

       This format statement would prepare records as follows:

       ±99__±99__±99__±999

    b. (I2,1X,I3,1X,2(I4,1X),I2) = ±9__±99__±999__±999__±9.

2. A decimal-oriented format statement

    A decimal number is indicated by an F. Two points must be considered. The first is the total number of characters in the number, including the decimal point. The second is the number of decimal places.

    a. (F11.4) = ±99999.9999

                       └──┘ *Number of decimal places = 4*

             └──────────┘ *Total width = 11*

    b. (3(F5.1,1X)) = ±99.9__±99.9__±99.9.

The program does not allow for the mixture of integers and decimals.

Section 6

Relationships Among Variates

Specific analyses of relationships have been described with Programs #22, #23, and #24. These analyses compare the alternatives of equal and non-equal cell frequencies.

The relationships between variates are first illustrated using the two-by-two table. The entries show two possibilities. In a) the frequencies are equal and denote no relationship; in b) there is massing of frequencies along the diagonal involving Row 1, Column 1, and Row 2, Column 2:

a) No Relationship

		Column		
Row	1	2	Total
1	10	10	20
2	10	10	20
Total	20	20	40

b) Positive Relationship

		Column		
Row	1	2	Total
1	20	0	20
2	0	20	20
Total	20	20	40

As one reads entry b from left to right, all of the observations are located in the smaller area for *both* measurements (Row and Column 1) and in the larger area for *both* measurements (Row and Column 2). This massing in the smaller and larger areas for both variates is called a positive relationship. That is, the variates show small values occurring together and large values together.

A *negative* or *inverse* relationship is the third possibility. Here, the massing is in Column 1, Row 2 (smaller values for the column variate are linked with larger values for the row variate) and in Column 2, Row 1. As the column values proceed from small to large, the row values proceed from large to small. The number of intervals defining the rows and columns are two in Program #22 and can be increased to a maximum of 10 in Program #23.

Program #25 Bivariate Plot

Another program used to consider and display relationships is the bivariate plot. This program provides the mechanism to define up to 1,000 cells accommodating up to 50 intervals on the row and up to 20 intervals on the column.

An example of the plot, with minima and maxima defined at program execution, is shown below. The number of observations in each cell is shown. Zero entries are not printed.

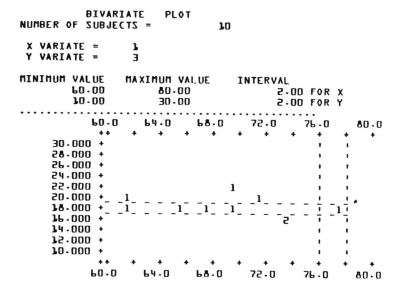

```
FOR X: GIVE MIN,MAX,NUMBER OF BOUNDARIES {MAX 21} ----?60,80,11

FOR Y: GIVE MIN,MAX,NUMBER OF BOUNDARIES {MAX 51} ----?10,30,11


              BIVARIATE    PLOT
NUMBER OF SUBJECTS =              10

X VARIATE =      1
Y VARIATE =      3

MINIMUM VALUE    MAXIMUM VALUE    INTERVAL
       60.00           80.00              2.00 FOR X
       10.00           30.00              2.00 FOR Y
. . . . . . . . . . . . . . . . . . . . . . . . . . . . . .
            60.0     64.0     68.0     72.0     76.0     80.0
            ++    +    +    +    +    +    +    +    +    +
   30.000 +                                   ¦    ¦
   28.000 +                                   ¦    ¦
   26.000 +                                   ¦    ¦
   24.000 +                                   ¦    ¦
   22.000 +                         1         ¦    ¦
   20.000 +_  _1_ _ _ _ _ _ _ 1_ _ _ _ _ _ ¦ _1¦_ ★
   18.000 +¯ _1_ _ _1_ _1_ _1_ _ _ _ _ _ ¦ _1¦¯
   16.000 +¯                        2¯ ¯ ¯ ¦¯  ¯
   14.000 +                                   ¦    ¦
   12.000 +                                   ¦    ¦
   10.000 +                                   ¦    ¦
            ++    +    +    +    +    +    +    +    +    +
            60.0     64.0     68.0     72.0     76.0     80.0
```

★ *One observation between 76 and 78 for the X variate and between 18 to 20 for the Y variate.*

In addition to this detailed table or graph, the program computes the relationship between the row variate (Y) and the column variate (X).

Note that the intervals for the Y variate decrease in value from top to bottom of the graph, while the intervals for the X variate increase from left to right. These changes in interval definitions also change the definition of positive and negative relationships.

A positive relationship now would be:

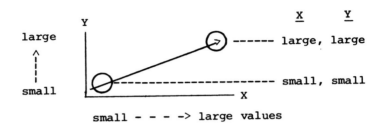

A negative relationship would be:

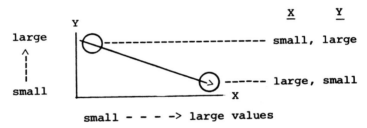

An analysis of the observations involves computation of the *regression line* describing the data. This is the line which comes "closest" to all of the observations.

The criterion used in finding the line is illustrated:

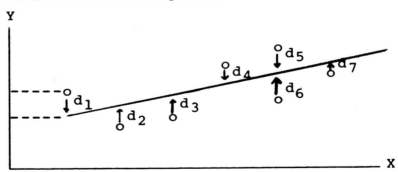

The distances from the observed data points (denoted by os) to the calculated regression line are indicated by $d_1, \ldots d_7$. These quantities, when squared and summed, must form the smallest total observed considering all possible lines describing these points. That line giving the smallest total is chosen as the regression line. This line is expressed in terms of its two parameters, A and B. The equation for a line is

$Y = A + B (X - \bar{X})$, where

X is the observed value of the measurement,

$\bar{X}$ is the mean value of the measurements,

A is the average value of the Y measurements, and

B is the slope of the line.

The slope expresses the change in Y for a constant change in X; that is,

$$B = \frac{Y_2 - Y_1}{X_2 - X_1} = \frac{Y_3 - Y_2}{X_3 - X_2}, \text{ etc.}$$

where the differences, $X_2 - X_1 = X_3 - X_2 \ldots$ etc., a constant interval length. The Y_1, Y_2, and Y_3 correspond to Y values at X_1, X_2, and X_3 respectively.

The program provides values of the confidence limits for the estimated line. These are given for the minimum, mean, and maximum values of the X variate. These confidence limit values are of use in deciding the emphasis to put on the line as an estimate of the relationship. Two examples are shown.

Wide limits:

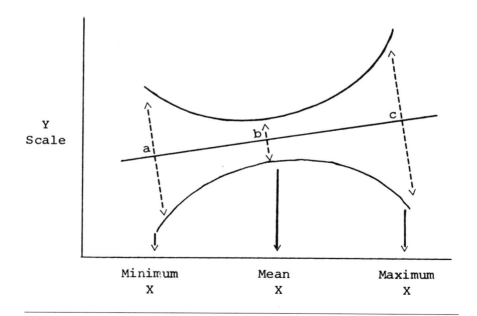

The distances at points a and c respectively may be quite large. The distance at b also may be large. The line may be the *best fit* of the observed values (criterion of smallest sum of squares) and yet be less than desirable as an estimate of the relationship between the X and Y variates.

Narrow limits:

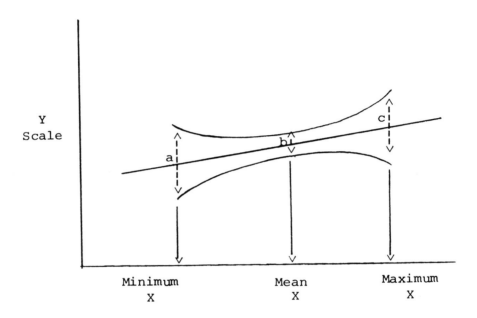

Y
Scale

Minimum
X

Mean
X

Maximum
X

Note that even at the widest points, a and c, the limits are "close together." At b, the limits almost touch the line. This situation suggests that the line would be a good estimator of the relationship between X and Y.

In both the wide and narrow limits examples, the limits were constructed using the same process. The construction method guarantees that, on repeated use with independent sets of data, a specified percent (the program allows for 95% or 99%) of the limits will include the *real* line which describes the relationship. The width of the limits depends upon the number of observations and the degree of variation among the points.

In addition to confidence limits for the line, confidence limits are reported describing an interval for the slope, B. If the interval contains the value zero, the regression line is not considered significant. If the interval does not include zero, the regression is significant.

Another statistic of value in judging the merits of the relationship is the *correlation coefficient.* This statistic is calculated and reported in Program #25. Values for the correlation coefficient range as follows:

+ 1—perfect positive relationship
0—no relationship
− 1—perfect negative relationship.

The correlation coefficient summarizes the information considered in calculating the line (distance of each point) and the direction of the relationship.

A convenient check on the analysis is provided by squaring the correlation coefficient. This number is the amount of variation (as a proportion) in the Y variate which may be *explained* by the line involving the X variate. For example:

Correlation Coefficient	Squared Value	Interpretation	
		Proportion of Y Variation Explained	
− 1.0	1.0		All variation explained
− 0.5	0.25	Negative Relationship	25% explained by X
− 0.2	0.04		4% explained by X
0	0		None explained
0.2	0.04		4% explained
0.5	0.25	Positive Relationship	25% explained
1.0	1.0		All variation explained

Frequently, correlations explaining 4% to 30% of the variation in the Y values are highly significant, even though the X variate used leaves from 70% to 96% (100% = percent squared correlation coefficient) unexplained. Interpreting significant regressions depends upon the degree of explanation considered satisfactory.

Program #27 Correlation Coefficients
All possible correlation coefficients among the variates taken in pairs may be calculated using Program #27. Significance testing may be performed using the tables provided in statistical texts. Identification of large correlation coefficients and squaring of these is a useful procedure for proper interpretation of relationships.

Correlation coefficients are used in many of the multivariate programs to establish relationships among the data. As considered here, any values of interest should be pursued using the bivariate plot program.

Summary

Programs analyzing relationships are structured to consider the degree of covariation between two variables. Variates with a small number of discrete values may be analyzed using Programs #22, #23, and #24. Variates with more values may be analyzed using Programs #25 or #27.

The primary objective is to determine if one of the two variates considered is related to the other in a way which shows that the information derived is *redundant*. If so, the more costly or more difficult to measure variate may be dropped with negligible loss in information.

Assessment of relationships improves with larger sample size and with a greater number of values describing the variate.

Index